# LOW CARB
## FOR THE BUSY, TIRED, ACHING, AND OVERWHELMED

An Easy-to-Digest Low Carb Guide to Reduce Pain, Inflammation, and Weight

Kristy Jo Wengert, FNS/WLS/CPT

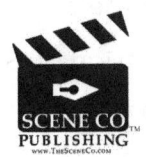

Copyright © 2020 by N8 and KJ Enterprises

All rights reserved. Published by Scene Co Publishing. No part of this book may be reproduced or transmitted in any form or by any means, electronic or otherwise, without written permission from the publisher.

Cover and title design by Shannon DeJong

ISBN 978-1-951411-05-3

www.thesceneco.com

To all of my Power Foods Lifestyle Champs:

*Thank you for allowing me to be a part of you and your family's lives.*

To find out more about the
Power Foods Lifestyle, please visit
www.PowerFoodsLifestyle.com

# TABLE OF CONTENTS

## Preparatory Chapters
Why Low Carb?........................................................1
  Important Carbohydrate Percentages Chart
Why Carbohydrates Matter........................................11
  Important Carbohydrate Samples Chart
Your Mindset Around Carbs....................................18

## How to Chapters
*Dive in here if you want to get started right away:*
Planning Your Meals..............................................22
Your Weekly To-Dos..............................................28
Meal Construction................................................32
Cooking Ideas.....................................................34
Grocery Shopping................................................41
Eating on the Road..............................................44
Beverages..........................................................48
Motivation.........................................................53

## Meal Plans:
Sample Meal Plans...............................................59
Sample Recipes...................................................70

# Chapter 1
# Why Low Carb?

In a world of conflicting opinions about food, where zealots defend the method of eating that works for *them*, and where digital media allows ads of all kinds to be placed in front of you after you look up a new recipe, it can be difficult at best to find a diet or nutritional practice that works for *you*.

I began coaching nutrition clients in 2013 and have watched in bewilderment as trends come and go in waves. Trainers, nutritionists, and doctors vacillate in their methods of teaching the general population what they should do with their food. I have spent a great deal of time in my profession dedicating myself to reviewing academic literature, new studies, podcasts, and books of other professionals to keep myself attuned with these trends.

I have been fortunate enough to have constant clientele to work with, and to have an open mind in working with each of these individuals. When working one-on-one with individuals, it is clear that nuance is present. No two individuals have the same set of circumstances, needs, or preferences. Adapting to those needs is one of the greatest markers for success. As the plan fits the individual, the individual is most likely to make the changes in their behavior to render improvements to their health, their management of pain, and even their body composition.

My nutrition methodology, The Power Foods Lifestyle (PFL), is, in itself, non-definitive. Instead, it is a structure of principles that can be applied in any combination to help individuals find the best nutritional approach for them. As I have taught and grown in my own anecdotal knowledge as a trainer and coach, as well as observed my colleagues and their own nutrition discoveries, my belief system in the Power Foods Lifestyle has grown and expanded as well.

> *Food must not hold morals in our mind.*

Additional principles, or the loosening of principles is fluid, and because I have seen so much change, I seek to hold no ego in a dictator-like approach toward food. The fact is, if it works for you, it works for you! Food must not hold morals in our mind. Rather, it is to be leveraged for the purpose of nourishing our bodies to the best they can be for our present conditions.

Currently, the Institute of Medicine proposes that Americans should obtain 45-65% of their calories from carbohydrates. As you read the next few chapters, I'd like you to ponder why this recommendation may not be ideal for everyone, especially you. I would also like you to ponder where extra carbohydrates may have been sneaking into your diet without you even being aware of it.

Let me now introduce to you why the low-carb strategy within the Power Foods Lifestyle is a fundamentally incredible method of eating for so many individuals. To do this, I'd first like to share why low-carb is important to me on a personal level.

At the age of 15, as a member of my high school drill team, I was doing a dance jump on the basketball floor where we practiced. I was drilling technique with 19 other girls on the drill team, and our coach was counting for us to complete the jump. Prep on 8, jump on 1. *Ready? 5, 6, 7, prep on 8, jump on 1!* Our coach wanted the synchronization to be seamless as we were dancing as one united team, even in practice.

After landing one of these jumps, I could not prepare for the next repetition. I felt paralyzed. My coach noticed I was unable to complete the jump with the rest of the group and yelled across the gymnasium, "What's going on, Kristy?" Completely in shock at the sizable 'zing' I had just felt all throughout my back, I couldn't respond, just started to cry. I couldn't move at all. Some of my teammates walked over to help me off the floor. My mom was called, and she drove me immediately to a chiropractic office, who happened to be a friend of the family. It was there I received the first X-ray of my back. As I viewed the 'S' shape curvature of my spine in black and white, I was told, "You have scoliosis."

*What? That's my back?!* I was floored. How did I not know my back was like that? I had always had a very flexible back in my dancing, doing movements that many of my teammates were jealous of... and now, here was the explanation. From that time forward, I began receiving electric muscle stimulation (EMS) in hopes of helping my spine begin to correct. The thought was that the concave parts of my spine had the strongest muscles, so needed to be weakened, and the elongated muscles on the convex portions of the curves needed to be strengthened to help push the spine back into straight alignment. In addition to this therapy, I also received spinal adjustments twice a week. This was all thanks to the generosity of this family friend, as my parents were not in a position to afford any more care for my back than this.

At the age of 22, I strongly considered having a rod put in my back to straighten my spine. But after doing a lot of research and talking to several individuals who had received the surgery, I opted out of surgery. By the time I graduated from college in 2011, I was in so much pain from dancing 4-6 hours each day that I was visiting an acupuncturist twice a week in addition to chiropractic and massage therapy.

My dream was to become an Artistic Director of dance at a university, and with a great deal of work and an intense audition, I was accepted to the University of Utah's Masters of Fine Arts program with an emphasis in modern dance. I'll never forget looking at that letter of acceptance and feeling pride surge within my heart.

My undergraduate degree was in English, yet I had been accepted to *this* program! That hardly ever happened, I was told by Dr. Li Lei, the artistic director of the university. And yet, in spite of achieving my goal, the next step to procuring the degree that would land me in my dream job, I knew I couldn't do it with the amount of pain I was in. How could I commit to another three years of dancing 4+ hours each day? I would never make it. So, I turned down the acceptance on the basis of fear of the unknown and what the time would do to my spine.

Indulge me to digress for a moment: Writing this now over a decade later, I still feel a surge of regret. At the time, I couldn't predict how my spine would handle the passing of time. At 33 years of age, currently, I now have the luxury of hindsight and an assurance of the condition of my spine. I now see that if I had gone forward with the program, I would have been able to complete the degree. With pain? Yes. But I would have been able to complete it.

Life is multi-dimensional. We make choices and we live with the consequences--both good and bad--with confidence. That is ownership, and something we will talk more about in the chapter on Mindset. I am taking ownership of this decision and believing it was the best choice I could have made--because without it, I would not be here writing this instruction book for you. The last decade of my life would have looked very different. I am grateful for all I have learned, experienced, and accomplished in that time through learning to set fierce goals, work through obstacles, and not allow fear and doubt to hold me down for too long. I am grateful for the life I have and am grateful dance has continued to remain in my life from teaching and coaching to judging and choreographing.

*My current goals for my spine are:*

1. Keep arthritis out by receiving regular chiropractic adjustments.
2. Keep inflammation (and consequently, pain) down through eating a low-carb PFL diet.
3. Keep moving and doing things I love to the best of my ability without flaring up in pain.

I believe that with these three points of action, I will live the best, fullest, and most productive life I can, in spite of living with chronic pain. Pain is my companion 24/7. One of the most important ways I can minimize the flare ups, achiness, and intensity of that pain is by reducing the carbohydrates in my diet. Other benefits that are helpful to note along the way include maintaining normal cholesterol and blood sugar levels, and having a leaner frame and body fat percentage. The latter additionally helps with pain as I am not carrying around as much weight on my asymmetrical bone structure.

## What Constitutes Low Carb?

Before I discuss the benefits of eating low-carb on a physiological level, I would first like to explain what constitutes a low-carb intake. The world has varying ideas of what low-carb is, for good reason. 'Low' to one person may be 'high' for another--it all depends on what a person is used to eating. A good portion of the nutrition world teaches that the way to define low-carb is through percentages of total macronutrient food intake between protein, carbohydrates, and fats.

1. Very low-carbohydrate (<10% carbohydrates)
2. Low-carbohydrate (<26% carbohydrates)
3. Moderate-carbohydrate (26%-44%)
4. High-carbohydrate (45% or greater)

But here is what drives me bonkers: the total caloric intake determines if these carb loads are actually hitting the desired target to reduce inflammation and pain. The target will be different for each person due to bio-individuality. Focusing on a percentage of our calories coming from carbs as our goal could ultimately lead us to think we are doing 'better' than we are. I don't recommend an individual tracks percentages alone, due to the fact that their total number of carbs per day may actually exit low-carb territory if their calories get high enough. That is why I teach a grams-per-day formula over percentages. I will explain this in more detail.

Power Foods Lifestyle Carb thresholds are defined by different ranges of daily carbohydrate intake. This allows the person to focus on total carbohydrates consumed, rather than on a titrating variable dependent on caloric intake.

1. Very low-carbohydrate (<35 grams of carbohydrates per day)
2. Low-carbohydrate (36-100 grams of carbohydrates per day)
3. Moderate-carbohydrate (101-170 grams of carbohydrates per day)
4. High-carbohydrate (171 grams of carbohydrates per day)

Study the table below to see the total daily grams of carbohydrates and how it changes depending on total caloric intake. You will see in the fourth column a few outliers that do not follow the pattern. Due to the higher calories, the range of carbs is higher than the previous line.

V-L-C: Very low-carbohydrate    L-C: Low-carbohydrate

M-C: Moderate-carbohydrate    H-C: High-carbohydrate

| Carbohydrate Percentage | Daily Calories | Carbohydrate Grams | PFL Carb Threshold |
|---|---|---|---|
| 5% | 1,500 | 18.75 g | V-L-C |
| 5% | 2,000 | 25 g | V-L-C |
| 5% | 2,500 | 31.25 | V-L-C |
| 10% | 1,500 | 37.5 g | L-C |
| 10% | 2,000 | 50 g | L-C |
| 10% | 2,500 | 62.5 | L-C |
| 20% | 1,500 | 75 g | L-C |
| 20% | 2,000 | 100 g | L-C |
| 20% | 2,500 | 125 g | M-C |
| 30% | 1,500 | 112.5 g | M-C |
| 30% | 2,000 | 150 g | M-C |
| 30% | 2,500 | 187.5 | H-C |
| 45% | 1,500 | 168.75 | M-C |
| 45% | 2,000 | 225 | H-C |
| 45% | 2,500 | 281.25 | H-C |

A few takeaways I would like to note from this table include:

1. Eating 1,500 calories with 10% of calories coming from carbohydrate is *not low enough* to constitute very-low-carb, or a ketogenic lifestyle.

2. The majority of women, when not actively managing their portions or food choices, will easily eat between 2,000 and 2,500 calories per day. *This means keeping carbohydrates at 20% will only qualify for a low-carb diet if she is eating fewer than 2,000 calories each day.*

3. Eating a lower-calorie diet of 1,500 and keeping carbs to 30% of the intake will *not be low enough to qualify for a low-carb diet*.

Having a higher percentage of carbohydrate intake like 45% with a lower-calorie diet of 1,500 calories can keep one in the moderate carb intake rather than high carbs.

In other words, it takes effort, strategy, and awareness to meet the criteria to qualify for a low-carb or very-low-carb method of eating. Most people who just 'wing it' won't actually push their carbs that low. This is one reason I recommend to my clients the tracking of their food in an app like *MyFitnessPal, CalorieCount,* or another app of their choice. This allows them to see their total daily grams in each of the three macronutrient groups (protein, carbs, and fats), rather than focusing only on percentages.

While tracking meticulously in this manner is not ideal for a sustainable lifestyle, it is *absolutely crucial* for aiming your intention, and training yourself as to what a complete day looks and feels like. Once you get this automaticity down, abandon your tracker and keep rolling with the principles and awareness you have gained. After some time passes, you might employ another 'dial-in' session of tracking to re-train your habits using numerical data.

> *While tracking meticulously... is not ideal for a sustainable lifestyle, it is absolutely crucial for aiming your intention.*

I also would like to acknowledge that for some populations, tracking can be problematic as it triggers an obsessiveness and compulsive behavior that leads to fear around foods. I was a part of this population from 2012-2015 following years of disordered eating and thinking. It took several years for me to retrain my mind and emotions around foods. *While it took patience and really learning about food by using the numbers, a breakthrough happened for me where food lost its morals of "good" or "bad" and, instead, I began to look at food as simply chemicals that would work differently in the 'engine' of my body.*

If you identify with being obsessed with foods, and worry about tracking for any amount of time, I urge you not to track—initially, at least. While tracking meticulously for as little as one week can help train yourself on portions and total macronutrient numbers, it is not worth it if this process triggers an infatuation or obsession that feels beyond the natural focus required for learning something new.

Instead, only focus on the PVF combination (a food from each of the categories Protein + Veggie + Fat I will explain later in the book) of foods principles outlined in this book. They are enough to lead you into a wonderful low-carb eating style. Considering a coaching session or two with me can also help you work around any fears or tendencies that may be holding you back. We will strategize together on the best approach for your psychology while meeting the physiological needs of low-carb. We are meant as human beings to be in community one with another. I enjoy listening to my clients' unique circumstances, helping them feel heard, and sharing insights, perspectives, and strategies that may help in their individual circumstances. If you would like to talk to me, you can contact me through my website.

## Net Carbs

The nuance of 'net carbs' is important for us as you have likely seen this phrase used on the label of food products in the grocery store. Net carbs are found when taking the total carbohydrates and subtracting the amount of dietary fiber and sugar alcohols. This is done due to common thought that fiber and sugar alcohols are not digested and absorbed, so have minimal effect on blood sugar.

However, buyer beware! Oftentimes, manufacturers include non-naturally occurring fiber to their product in order to decrease the carbohydrates, allowing them to market a 'lower-carb' product. In actuality, these types of products often still impact blood sugar.

Due to all I have observed, the Power Foods Lifestyle principle for net carbs remains as follows:

- If more than 15% of your daily food intake comes from processed foods, I do not recommend counting net carbs. Count the total +carbohydrates in your foods to assess if you are getting your carbohydrates to a low-carb threshold of 36-100 grams of carbohydrates per day.

- If fewer than 15% of your daily food intake comes from processed foods, meaning the majority of the foods you eat are unprocessed power foods, I recommend counting net carbs. Decrease the total grams of fiber (though not sugar alcohols) from the total carbohydrate count to arrive at your daily net carbohydrates.

I have chosen not to include net carbs in any of the meal plans or recipes I create. You may wish to calculate the net carbs from these, if you desire for your specific situation.

## Will You Benefit from Low Carb?

Along with the reasons I personally benefit from a low-carb diet, there are many more demographics of people I have witnessed that benefit from a low-carb strategy. While this list is non-exhaustive, it may help give you an idea if this approach* might be right for you:

- » Alzheimer's Disease
- » Arthritis
- » Bipolar Disorder
- » Brain Injury

- Chronic Pain
- Epilepsy
- Depression**
- Fibromyalgia
- Hypothyroidism
- Insulin Resistance
- Multiple Sclerosis
- Non-alcoholic Fatty Liver Disease
- Overweight
- Parkinson's Disease
- PCOS
- High Blood Sugar
- High Blood Pressure
- High Cholesterol
- Type 2 Diabetes

\* Please check with your health care provider before changing your diet, particularly if you are on medications. Each individual's dietary needs are unique. You are ultimately responsible for all decisions which impact your health.

\*\* This includes postpartum depression, but only if the mother is not breastfeeding, as more carbohydrates are generally needed for milk production.

# Chapter 2: Why Carbohydrates Matter

Before I begin a brief science lesson, I would like you to be aware of where carbohydrates generally come from. Take a moment to look at the table below, where I have included some basic categories of foods that are known to have carbs in them. I have included a few common foods with their macronutrient breakdown. Notice the amount of carbs in a serving of each item and how the grams of carbs go lower the further down the chart we get.

\* Each number in this chart is in units of grams and are rounded to the nearest gram.

\*\* p = protein, c = carbohydrate, f = fat

| SUGARY SNACKS | | | |
|---|---|---|---|
| *This is a VERY RARELY EAT category for Carbs in your low-carb Lifestyle.* | | | |
| Chocolate Chip Cookie (small) | 3 p | 36 c | 12 f |
| Starburst Candies (8 candies) | 0 p | 34 c | 3 f |
| Cinnamon Toast Crunch Cereal (1 cup) | 1 p | 32 c | 5 f |
| SUGARY DRINKS | | | |
| *This is a VERY RARELY DRINK category for Carbs in your low-carb Lifestyle* | | | |
| Chocolate Milk (1 cup) | 8 p | 26 c | 9 f |
| Orange Juice (1 cup) | 2 p | 26 c | 1 f |
| Apple Juice (1 cup) | 1 p | 28 c | 0 f |

| GRAINS | | | |
|---|---|---|---|
| *This is a VERY RARELY EAT category for Carbs in your low-carb Lifestyle.* | | | |
| Whole Grain Bread (2 slices) | 12 p | 34 c | 4 f |
| Original Bagel (½ bagel) | 7 p | 37 c | 2 f |
| Penne Pasta (1 cup cooked) | 4 p | 22 c | 1 f |
| STARCHY VEGETABLES | | | |
| *This is an OCCASIONALLY EAT category for Carbs in your low-carb Lifestyle.* | | | |
| Sweet Potato (4 oz.) | 2 p | 24 c | 0 f |
| Red Potato (4 oz.) | 2 p | 19 c | 0 f |
| Butternut Squash (4 oz.) | 1 p | 14 c | 0 f |
| SWEET FRUITS | | | |
| *This is an OCCASIONALLY EAT category for Carbs in your low-carb Lifestyle.* | | | |
| Pineapple (½ cup) | 0 p | 11 c | 0 f |
| Banana (½ medium) | 1 p | 14 c | 0 f |
| Mango (½ cup) | 1 p | 12 c | 0 f |
| BERRIES | | | |
| *This is a SOMETIMES EAT category for Carbs in your low-carb Lifestyle.* | | | |
| Strawberries (½ cup) | 1 p | 8 c | 0 f |
| Blueberries (½ cup) | 1 p | 11 c | 0 f |
| Raspberries (½ cup) | 1 p | 7 c | 0 f |
| CRUCIFEROUS VEGGIES | | | |
| *This is a DAILY EAT category for Veggies in your low-carb Lifestyle.* | | | |
| Broccoli (1 cup) | 3 p | 6 c | 0 f |
| Cauliflower (1 cup) | 2 p | 5 c | 0 f |
| Brussels Sprouts (1 cup) | 2 p | 7 c | 0 f |
| LEAFY GREENS | | | |
| *This is a DAILY EAT category for Veggies in your low-carb Lifestyle.* | | | |
| Spinach (1 cup raw) | 1 p | 1 c | 0 f |
| Arugula (1 cup raw) | 1 p | 1 c | 0 f |
| Chard (1 cup raw) | 1 p | 1 c | 0 f |

While there are differing types of sugar, like lactose (dairy products) and fructose (fruits), the body breaks down and converts most carbohydrates into glucose. For the sake of simplicity, we will refer to all sugars as carbs in this instruction book.

Carbohydrates that start out as glucose begin digesting the moment they enter your mouth, with the enzyme amylase in your saliva. A healthy body functions to utilize those sugars in different ways. While these conversations can become very complex, I like to keep things simple, so let's break down their role into three parts:

1. Fuel the Brain
2. Fuel the Muscles
3. Storage for Lack of Glucose

Glucose fuels the brain with energy as well as the muscles with energy. If that energy is needed right away, sugar is pulled into the cells by way of the hormone insulin, and then the glucose is readily available. This is what happens in the case of the person who just went jogging, then refueled with some carbohydrate food or drink for more energy, or the mom who ran errands all day, felt a blood sugar drop resulting in weakness, shakiness, and a headache, then ate some carbohydrates to regulate that blood sugar. This is a common mechanism of eating and often happens without us thinking much about it other than, "I need some food because I feel weak."

In a healthy individual, insulin is secreted from the pancreas to get the glucose out of the blood and into the cells to be used. If there is any extra sugar that is not actively needed by the brain or muscles, it is stored in the muscle sites and liver until they are full. Glucose is stored in the form of glycogen, where the glucose is strung together into a long chain until it is needed by the body in a future shortage of sugar. If that happens, another hormone, glucagon, begins the breakdown of glycogen to get sugar back into the blood for the cells to utilize and shuttle energy to the muscles and brain. The liver and muscle sites have been found to hold an average of 500 grams of glucose.

DID YOU KNOW THIS ABOUT SUGAR AND THE SCALE? *It takes water to store glucose as glycogen. This is one reason why you should not be overly alarmed at a rise in scale weight if you have eaten more carbohydrates within 24 hours before weighing. Depending on how much carbohydrate you currently had in storage, and the amount you just ate (assuming a healthily-functioning insulin response), you did not gain body fat. Your glucose reserves are simply holding that extra sugar with water as glycogen. This simple fact has helped many of my clients who are very aware of their weight to step away from emotional tail-spins that happen when trying to eat better but don't see a drop in their weight right away. Your body can fluctuate 5-8 pounds just based on carbohydrate storage and water intake alone! While my goal in this instruction book is not to get too much into shifting body composition, weight loss may absolutely occur when shifting to a low-carb nutnutrition strategy.*

Unfortunately, insulin resistance is becoming a very common condition in America. Due to poor eating habits with large amounts of consumption of refined, processed foods with added sugars, many Americans experience an impaired sensitivity of the cells to insulin. Therefore, they do not allow glucose into the cells to be used for energy. Instead, glucose is shuttled away to be stored as fat because that sugar must do *something*. Insulin is a storage hormone, so if the cells do not take the sugar away, insulin will do its job and pack it away--usually in our stomach, hips, inner thighs, and buttocks. I am not writing this book to discuss *how* insulin resistance occurs, but rather, *what to do if you notice you have this condition along with any of the others I have listed above.*

You may be wondering how your brain and muscles can function if you don't have a full supply of carbohydrates? Your body was designed to handle this situation beautifully, which is why PFL low-carb is a nutrition strategy we can use to our benefit for certain demographics.

In a shortage of incoming glucose, the liver calls upon another metabolic pathway by producing a secondary fuel called ketones. These ketones cross the blood-brain barrier and make up for the deficient glucose. (In our PFL low-carb method of eating, you will still be getting *some* glucose--not pushing that glucose *extremely* low like a Keto diet, but you will also not be getting an *abundant* amount.) Refer back to V-L-C, L-C, etc. in the table in *Why Low Carb?*

As for exercise, a slower, yet more efficient method of fueling the muscles than burning glucose is by breaking down adipose tissue for fatty acids. Fatty acids provide steady energy to the muscles for most exercise that stays in an aerobic state. An aerobic state means you are not pushing to extremely high heart rates, keeping to 60-75% of maximum heart rate. Higher heart rates than this are best fueled by carbohydrates.

As you can see, the body has simple methods of compensating when glucose is in lower supply. Your brain and muscles will not suffer but will adapt to the different methods of being fueled. This adaptation process can take anywhere from 3-14 days, but once your body adjusts, you should feel vibrant and sustained in energy.

Again, *I am not teaching you a Keto diet.* Keto's primary goal is to help your body function 100% off ketones for energy rather than glucose by getting the carbs low enough for a Very Low-Carb strategy. While a low-carb eating approach will generate ketones to supplement incoming glucose, the goal is not to switch to a fat-fueled environment only. This instruction book is for a low-carb nutrition strategy.

If you wish to learn a Keto strategy and feel it is the next step for you after trying the low-carb approach from the *Power Foods Lifestyle*, check out PowerFoodsLifestyle.com to see if my PFL Keto Course is available.

## Inflammation

The food you eat influences the makeup of the billions of gut microbes that comprise your microbiome. The microbiome composition has been found in recent research to be responsible for many of the health conditions we individually experience, including mental health disorders. Your microbiome composition is constantly changing due to the foods and beverages you ingest, environmental toxins, pollution, topical toxins, and anything else that goes into or onto your body.

Carbohydrates, particularly those in the grains and refined sugars category I call 'non-strategic carbs,' have been found to encourage the growth of inflammatory gut bacteria. Because of the interaction of the gut and immune system (which lines the gut), the state of the microbiome is critical for how the immune system's defense functions. If your body has more inflammatory gut bacteria, you will experience more pain in your body.

Inflammation is the body's immune response to toxins in the body as it works to purify itself. The more toxins enter your body, the more biochemical responses engage. Inflammation often manifests as pain or aggravation of a host of possible health symptoms. The fewer toxins you put in your body, the less inflammation you experience. A lowered inflammatory response may also help with side effects that frequently occur from taking medications.

Simply stated, when you eat healthy power foods with minimal sugar, grains, or processing, you feed your gut bacteria and help it grow stronger and more productive. This healthy microbiome interacts less frequently with the immune system because there are fewer toxins present (at least in the foods and beverages you ingest). This lower frequency interaction leads to less inflammation, resulting in less exaggeration of pain, symptoms of other health conditions, and feeling 'yucky' all around.

## Weight Loss

While this book is primarily focused on reducing pain, inflammation, and flare-ups from chronic conditions, weight loss may occur as well when transitioning to a low-carb nutritional approach. Weight loss may be a helpful part of your pain management plan. To lose weight, I recommend tracking your calories and total grams of carbohydrates to ensure you are in a caloric deficit. That is the simple biomechanics of energy balance. When you eat less than you burn, you will lose weight. In addition to the caloric deficit, managing your total carbohydrate intake will help reduce the inflammation in your body.

However, you do not need to track calories to get wonderful results. As you listen to your body to be mindful and aware of hunger and fullness cues, you may be able to put yourself in a caloric deficit without meticulously tracking. As you choose your meals, mind the PVF strategy I will outline soon in this book. The general hypothesis around why you can easily lose weight while on a low-carb strategy is this: more focus on eating fat and protein increases your satisfaction after a meal. The focus on these two macronutrient groups additionally produces less vacillation of blood sugar, which leads to a greater frequency of being in a fat burn zone (I explain this in detail in my book, *The Power Foods Lifestyle, Edition 2*).

There is also a theory that eating more protein and fat, and fewer carbohydrates, in a day leads to an increase in thermogenesis (utilization of fat for energy), with approximately 200-300 more calories burned naturally per day as compared to a moderate to high-carb intake diet. This theory remains controversial but is interesting to note. Soon enough, you will be able to see for yourself if you can feel a difference in your body without being part of a study group.

## Let's Get to Work

As you learn the how-to's of minimizing the carbs you eat, and focusing on *intentional eating* using proteins (P), vegetables (V), and fats (F), you will be able to experiment for yourself and learn of the benefits through experience. Give the PFL low-carb strategy a solid two weeks of effort with no expectations. You won't feel a difference overnight in most cases--it takes time for your body to adapt! But trust me—the time will come you DO feel a difference. So keep going and look forward to your body's manifestations that you are doing something wonderful for it. I'm so excited for you to enjoy the benefits of the PFL low-carb strategy!

# Chapter 3:
# Your Mindset Around Carbs

It is crucial to be mindful of your thoughts around carbohydrates. In this section, I'd like to encourage you to challenge the beliefs and feelings you have around carbs of all types.

Each of us has a set of beliefs around foods. These beliefs come from our environment, the people we're around, the literature we read, and the marketing we see.

> *Each of us has a set of beliefs around food.*

As you learn to condition your mind toward a 'food is fuel' and 'nutrition strategy' over a 'diet mentality,' you will begin to breathe in this low-carb lifestyle and find it truly fitting for you. It takes time, so do not be discouraged if it doesn't feel like it's freeing you from your pain or other symptoms for a time.

John Allen, author of *As a Man Thinketh*, pens ideals about the power of thought so profoundly that I have often had to stop and ponder one of his quotes for a full day. I'd like to provide you with three of his most profound statements to me on thought. (And yes, we ladies can replace 'man' with 'woman.' This language is fitting for the time and not gender exclusive).

1. "A man is literally what he thinks, his character being a complete sum of all his thoughts."

2. "A man is but the product of his thoughts. What he thinks, he becomes."

3. "As you think, you travel and as you love, you attract. You are today where your thoughts have brought you; you will be tomorrow where your thoughts take you."

Learn to be aware of, define, and direct your thoughts around food. Be mindful of, and explore the potential for, your low-carb lifestyle and your body's capabilities. Invite into your mind the belief in your ability to follow through on actions that are beneficial for you. As you seek to do this daily, you will easily be able to meet your goals.

## Let's Define Carbohydrates

There are different types of carbs that we can group into three categories:

Veggie Carbs: Vegetables that are not starchy (this excludes potatoes, pumpkins, and large squash) that are grown naturally from the earth and contain fewer than 8 grams of total carbohydrates per cup. Veggie carbs are typically much lower in how they impact your blood sugar due to their higher concentration of fiber. Examples of veggie carbs include broccoli, zucchini, asparagus, celery, cucumber, spinach, and arugula.

Power Carbs: Carbohydrates that are much denser in carbohydrates and can also be starchy. These are grown naturally from the earth and typically contain between 10-30 grams of carbohydrates per ½-1 cup. Power carbs, while healthier and containing needed fiber, still impact blood sugar to some degree. Examples of power carbs include oats, sweet potatoes, beans, rice, wheat, lentils, apples, berries, and grapefruit.

Non-Strategic Carbs: Carbohydrates that do not grow in natural settings and tend to be high in both carbs and fats. Any food or beverage with refined or added sugars, extra processing, or non-natural ingredients belongs in this category. These carbs usually lack much nutrient density, meaning the vitamins and minerals per calorie are extremely low. If you are experiencing any condition I mentioned in Chapter 1, this category of carbs is one to stay away from as much as possible. Non-strategic carbs will incite inflammation in your body. Examples of non-strategic carbs include ice cream, candy, brownies, cookies, bagels, white pasta, and crackers.

Now, for a touchier topic before we dive into the logistics of your low-carb lifestyle:

You may have heard eating low-carb for too long could impact your thyroid function, decrease testosterone, and even raise cortisol. While this can circumstantially be true, remember that all nutritional studies try to find generalized conclusions. It is impossible to find and define every unique nuance of demographic, portion size, activity level, gender, and genetic profile in any given study. There is simply not enough time, researchers, or funding to cover it all. So, we take that research with a grain of salt and, after doing an initial 2-4 week test period of low-carb eating, decide where your body functions best. Do not let generalized research where *correlations* may be found lead you to believe you should not do something great for your health because you believe it's as good as causation. Correlation and causation are two completely separate relationships.

Intuition plus experimentation with PFL strategies leads to personalized solutions. I believe that if you eat in a way that feels right to your body based on 1) the management of symptoms, 2) enjoyment and sustainability, and 3) nourishment and function of bodily processes, you will be led to the level of carbohydrate intake right for *your body.*

Just like my story of turning down my graduate degree of dance, based on *fear of the unknown*, it can be easy for us to turn down a wonderful future. Be aware that in this world of so much information overload due to technology, you can easily stumble across a piece of research or an article that motivates you away from what you come to think and feel about nutrition. I encourage you to read any nutrition information, including the information I am sharing with you, with a mindset to go with what feels intrinsically right to you.

While it is important to filter through information to find what feels right to you, it can be too easy to discard life-changing information. If you will listen to one voice at a time and eliminate the noise in your life, you will discover the perfect low-carb strategy that is right for you. Let this instruction book be your starting point to get the ball rolling, then let's see where you end up as you listen to your body. I can't wait to hear of your success!

# Chapter 4:
# Planning Your Meals

Planning your meals is the most fundamental part of a low-carb lifestyle. While in-depth planning for an initial two to six-week training period is fundamental, a heightened level of awareness and planning may not be sustainable. Your goal should be to eventually get to a point where you can just "wing it" based on the habits you have developed. I believe that when you implement a simple, yet flexible structure to your meals each week, you will feel more at ease. I will teach you how to develop that structure in this chapter. Your mind will not be consumed by food all day long as you practice and work the system. You will feel confident that this is a lifestyle you can easily stick with.

There are four basic food groups I would like you to use to describe foods: proteins, carbohydrates, fats, and veggies. The first three are often referred to as 'macros.' All foods' calories are divided up into these macro categories as the grams of proteins, carbohydrates, and fats contribute the total caloric amount. While veggies are technically carbohydrates, they're much lower in comparison to other carbs, so we put them in their own category. A simple way to look at this is to remember any vegetable classified should be less than 10 grams of carbohydrates per cup serving. If it is more than that, it goes in the carb category. An interesting part of the Power Foods Lifestyle is that I, in other strategies, I help individuals start to systematize their portions of Carbohydrates using a 20-30 gram measurement. This applies whether they are choosing a power carb or a non-strategic carb. Over time, I like to see more and more of their carb choices come from power carb foods. As you follow the PFL low-carb strategy, I would like you to be mindful of this. While it is not wise to eat non-strategic carbs, if you do, it is better to portion them out than to swing to the extreme of saying you just can't do the lifestyle. Start where you're at, and optimize from there. As you work on your new low-carb strategy, you will predominantly only choose veggie carbs (V) to accompany protein and fat-based foods to make a PVF meal.

It is important that you learn which macro group basic foods belong to. This makes meal construction and food pairing very easy once you get the hang of this system. Take a look at the following lists to see some basic classifications. As you gain experience, you can begin determining on your own which category a food belongs to:

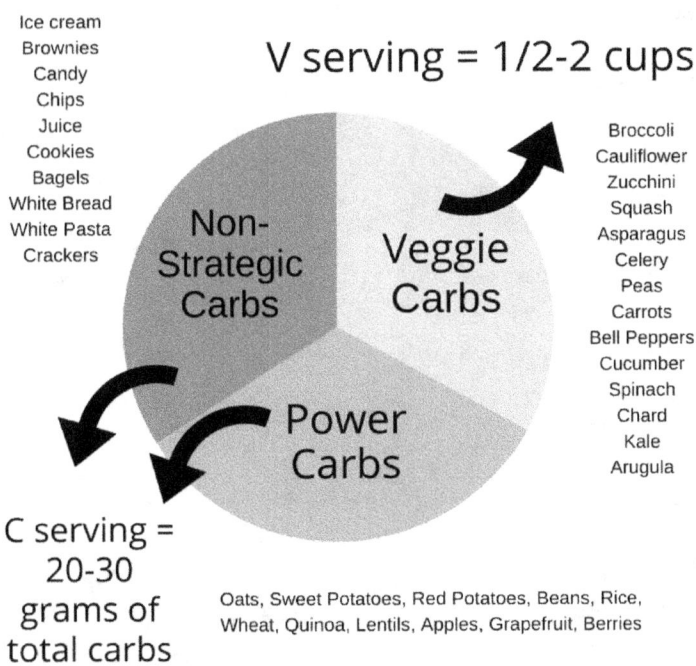

Proteins (P):

    Chicken Breast
    Cottage Cheese
    Egg Whites
    Ground Turkey
    Ground Beef*
    Protein Powder
    Salmon

*Important note: The Power Foods Lifestyle principle is to eat red meat only 1-3x/week. Not too infrequently as your body needs the CLA (Conjugated Linoleic Acid), B12, and iron, but also not so frequently as red meat, in abundance, can also trigger an inflammatory response.*


Carbs (C):

    Apples
    Berries
    Beans
    Brown Rice
    Chickpeas
    Grapefruit
    Lentils
    Red Potato
    Sweet Potato


Fats (F):

    Almonds
    Avocado
    Cashews
    Chia Seeds
    Coconut Oil
    Egg Yolks
    Olives
    Olive Oil
    Pumpkin Seeds

Of course, there is so much nuance to foods. Many people are surprised, for example, that beans and lentils are actually carbs instead of proteins. This goes for nuts and cheese being fats instead of protein as well. I explain this in detail in my main book, *The Power Foods Lifestyle, Edition 2*. If you would like a thorough explanation of how to determine which food falls under which category, please check out that book next. Your life will be enriched by learning about these deeper systems of becoming a master of how you look at food.

You can achieve the goal of having a low-carb meal without leaving out other important nutrients through a simple strategy. This meal strategy is called PVF meals. PVF = Protein-Veggie-Fat. Simply choose a food from each of these three categories and make a meal of it. You can also choose more than one food from each category. You can choose to have small servings of each of these foods (if eating 4-6 meals per day) or you can choose larger portions of these foods (if eating 1-3 meals per day).

## Simple PVF meals:

>PF: Whole Eggs (the egg yolk is a fat)
>V: Spinach
>*Cooking: Use non-stick spray to scramble the spinach and eggs together. Season with salt and pepper to taste.*

>P: Chicken Breast
>V: Broccoli
>F: Avocado
>*Cooking: Pressure cook the chicken in a pressure cooker and shred with two forks. Steam broccoli and add freshly sliced avocado. Season with salt and pepper to taste.*

P: Cottage Cheese
V: Cucumber
F: Almonds
*Preparation: Dice the cucumber into the Cottage Cheese and add almonds. For flavor, add sea salt, pepper, salsa, or even Ranch powder mix and stir in well.*

If you are counting calories, I advise you to keep to simple PVF structure so your meals have less food and caloric volume. However, if you're not as worried about counting calories and simply trust your "fullness meter" to tell you how much is too much, the complex PVF method below may be more enjoyable for you. This method should be done if eating 4 or fewer meals per day.

## Complex PVF meals:

PF: Whole Eggs (the egg yolk is a fat)

V: Spinach
V: Bell Pepper
F: Coconut Oil
F: Shredded Cheese
*Cooking: Sauté the bell pepper and spinach in oil. Scramble the eggs and cheese in. Season with salt and pepper to taste.*

P: Chicken Breast
V: Broccoli
V: Asparagus
V: Mushrooms
F: Avocado
F: Olive Oil
*Cooking: Pressure cook the chicken in the Instant Pot and shred with two forks. Sauté all of the chopped veggies in olive oil. Add freshly sliced avocado. Season with salt and pepper to taste.*

P: Cottage Cheese
P: Turkey Breast
V: Cucumber
V: Celery
F: Almonds
F: Olives

*Preparation: Dice the veggies and turkey breast into the Cottage Cheese. Add almonds and sliced olives. For flavor, add sea salt, pepper, salsa, or even Ranch powder mix and stir in well.*

*This book* is strictly a how-to manual, which leads me to provide a basic sound bite for each macronutrient so you remember why it is important. In *The Power Foods Lifestyle, Edition 2*, I go into *deep detail* about the health benefits and properties of proteins, carbs, fats, and veggies. Below are simple refreshers from those chapters:

*Protein:* Anchors the blood sugar, helps the body rebuild millions of cells each new day, and supports lean muscle tissue.

*Carbohydrates:* Provide energy to the brain and muscles--but in this low-carb eating book, we learn to rely on more fats for energy

*Fats:* An energy source that helps your body absorb crucial vitamins A, E, D, and K, as well as signal your body to release a hormone called Cholecystokinin, which tells your body you are full after eating a meal.

*Vegetables:* Provide your body with essential vitamins, minerals, and fiber which keep your body and brain functioning properly.

# Chapter 5:
# Your Weekly To-Dos

As you embrace this new lifestyle, there are some weekly tasks you can do to best set yourself up for success.

## Make a Grocery List Each Week

Set a weekly alarm in your phone or recurring appointment in your digital calendar to remind you to do your meal planning and grocery shopping. Do this at the same time each week for more automatic behaviors that become a way of life for you.

For the first few weeks of learning the power foods, use the list at the end of this book to select 4-5 foods from each of the four categories: protein, veggies, carbs, and fats. It can be too easy to become overzealous and buy a ton of produce that you will not use before it goes bad. Not only is this overwhelming when you go to look in the fridge, but this is why the 4-5 foods per category per week process works remarkably well. If you get the hang of it after a month or so, you should definitely expand that list so you get even more variety of nutrients, but in portions that you know you will use and never waste.

When selecting the 4-5 foods, select those you are already familiar with cooking and eating. If this nutrient-dense lifestyle is *very* new for you, I'm going to ask you to be brave and try foods that you may have previously thought you didn't like. In the next chapter on cooking, I'll be sharing my simple cooking methods most of my trainees have raved about. Most who have tried my food over the years end up being surprised, *even when they previously thought they didn't like a food.*

## Brainstorm Your Meals for the Week

It's one thing to get the right foods in your house, but the next level is knowing what you're going to make! If you leave it to the moment you are ready to eat, you may not come up with the best option. The individuals I have worked with have always excelled and made a sustainable lifestyle for themselves when they have a simple paper posted on the fridge for the week with a few ideas for meals.

It is usually easiest to have two ideas for breakfast, lunch, and snacks, while having five ideas for dinner. If you are making enough for leftovers each day, lunch can easily be yesterday's leftovers. By only planning five dinners, you leave room for unforeseen events, trips away from home, or people coming over with food (plus, it's never a bad idea to repeat a meal from earlier in the week!).

Here is a sample of what your meal planning paper can look like:

| Breakfast | Lunch | Snacks | Dinner |
| --- | --- | --- | --- |
| 1. | 1. | 1. | 1. |
| 2. | 2. | 2. | 2. |
|  |  |  | 3. |
|  |  |  | 4. |
|  |  |  | 5. |

## Meal Prep

As you might see on Instagram under the hashtag #FoodPrep, meal preparation may look like a spread of every single meal made in advance and portioned into perfect containers. While this method of preparation can be helpful for very busy people, it is not required to succeed in a new eating strategy. As I have coached thousands of people over the past eight years, I have discovered the greater majority of people do better with a 'piece-meal' food prep. I recommend doing this form of preparation twice a week. I tend to do this on a Sunday for Monday, Tuesday, and Wednesday's meals, then another prep on Wednesday for Thursday, Friday, and Saturday's meals. Sunday tends to be a catch-up day where I have more time to use whatever is left in the fridge to make meals.

Here is what a piece-meal prep using some basic foods you buy for the week. If you do not see a food on this list, I haven't found a sustainable way to prepare it so just cut it up or cook it on the same day you will eat it. Of course, you can and should cook in bulk, or at least enough for there to be leftovers for the next day.

Veggies:

- » Bell Peppers: Wash and dice/slice and put in a container for up to three days.
- » Onion: Dice and put in a container for up to one week.
- » Cucumbers: Wash, but only slice fresh on the day of use.
- » Leafy Greens: Wash, pat dry, and chop. Put in a container for up to three days or place in an air-tight Ziplock bag with no moisture for up to five days.
- » Zucchini/Squash: Wash and dice/slice and put in a container for up to two days.
- » Carrots: Wash and slice and put in a Ziplock baggie for up to four days.
- » Broccoli: wash well and slice into small florets. Place in a Ziplock baggie for up to four days.
- » Celery: Wash and slice and put in a container or Ziplock baggie for up to four days.
- » Tomatoes: Wash and dice and put in a container for up to three days.

Meat:

- » Chicken: Cube or place as a breast in individual Ziplock bags. You can bulk cook chicken in the Instant Pot or crockpot, shred, and keep in the refrigerator for up to three days.

- » Beef: Section out 3-4 ounces of beef into individual Ziplock bags. Smash flat and freeze until the day you will use it. Browned beef keeps in the fridge for up to three days.

- » Fish: If purchasing fresh, section out 3-4 ounce filets and freeze in individual Ziplock bags. Cook fish only on the day you plan to eat it.

Planning your meals is the antidote to anxiety and overthinking your nutrition. With simple ideas and a simple meal construction process (PVF or PVFc (lower-case 'c' representing a smaller portion of power carbs, about the size of a small fist)), you can easily make the right nutrition happen for your body, reduce pain and inflammation, and do so without needing to be an expert of nutrition or even cooking.

# Chapter 6:
# Meal Construction

You may be wondering how much of a food makes a proper portion. This is a very nuanced conversation, but I will try to make it as easy for you as possible.

In *The Power Foods Lifestyle Edition 2*, I discuss how eating 6 small meals per day is an optimal eating pattern. One of the main reasons behind this is it allows us to get extremely descriptive in proper portions for protein, fats, and carbs because we understand how many meals will go in the day. When we don't operate on a standard number of meals per day, it becomes a bit trickier to do this, though it is still absolutely doable.

In this low-carb strategy book, I'd like to discuss more of a general approach that will help you get a great starting point. From there, listen to your body and hunger cues. Sometimes it takes a week or two to regulate hunger signals, as well as recognize fullness, if we have really been off our nutrition game for a while. Be patient with yourself during this process. Consider the portion sizes listed below to get started. You will need a food scale initially to train yourself on the weight of food until your eyes can easily recognize the proper portion for yourself.

*Please note: The portions I generally teach are for semi-active women who are looking to eat 1,400-1,600 calories per day. This usually puts a female in a slight caloric deficit to lose a bit of body fat in a sustainable way. If you would like more calories than this, I recommend making the portion sizes a bit larger. Above all, listen to your body if you are trying to simply maintain weight, but feel better by eating more strategically in this low-carb strategy.*

| Food | Weigh/Measure It | Eyeball It |
|---|---|---|
| Meat | 3-4 ounces per serving | The size of a deck of cards |
| Yogurt/Cottage Cheese | ½-¾ cup per serving | A small fist |
| Leafy Greens | 2 cups chopped | 2 large handfuls |
| Most Veggies | 1-2 cups chopped | 2 large handfuls |
| Nuts/Seeds | ½-1 ounce | A large palmful |
| Olives | ½ cup | A handful |
| Cheese | 1 ounce | A large palmful |
| Rice/Beans/Couscous | ½ cup cooked | A small fist |
| Red/Sweet Potatoes | 2-3 ounces | A small fist |
| Fruit | ½ cup | A small fist |

## Remember the Simple Meal Structure:

PV (Protein-Veggie) = the anchor to every meal

F (Fat) = the energy to a meal

C (Carbs) = *power carbs are okay in small amounts, but other carbs will bring about inflammation to your body that is not helpful for demographics searching for less pain and more freedom in their bodies.*

Therefore, the meals you will eat from here on out will be a PVF and once in a while, you will eat a PVFc. The lower-case 'c' refers to a smaller portion of carbohydrates than a typical 20-30 grams. A half portion would be 10-15 grams of total carbs.

For the first two weeks of your low-carb power foods approach, I encourage you to abstain from any power or non-strategic carbs at all. After week two, explore some of the power carbs in small portions. In this new period of creating your low-carb lifestyle, listen to your body. Pain, discomfort, bowel movement disruption, or other symptoms will let you know if more or less carb amounts per day is right for you. You can view different suggestions for PVF and PVFc meals in the Sample Recipes and Meal Plan chapters at the end of the book.

# Chapter 7:
# Cooking Ideas

Whether you feel you are fabulous or a flop in the kitchen, you will excel at this low-carb lifestyle when you remember the five S's.

1. Salad
2. Scramble
3. Shake
4. Soup
5. Stir-fry

You may not be making the routine meals you are accustomed to, or what our society has led you to believe is a customary meal for breakfast, lunch, or dinner. Instead, you get to craft a new lifestyle that will have you confidently create your meals in a balanced, anti-inflammatory, and freedom-based way.

Using the five S's will help you take any PVF or PVFc-based foods to create something great! All you will need is to add some good seasonings or sauces, then you will have simple, delicious, balanced meals that are not only nutritious and helpful for managing pain and chronic conditions, but will help you shed excess weight too if desired.

*Here are a few examples to get your creative juices flowing:*

1. For this first example, let's go with Salmon (PF) + Asparagus (V) + Avocado Oil (F).

*Salad:* Bake the salmon. Cube and place over a bed of leafy greens (it's okay to add another V, especially when it's a salad). Steam the asparagus and put on top of the salad, then drizzle with avocado oil for dressing. Be sure to add any other veggies you'd like to add color, like tomatoes, orange bell peppers, or mushrooms.

*Scramble:* Follow the directions for stir-fry below, but then add liquid egg whites (½ cup) or full eggs (2 eggs=PF) to scramble it up and add extra protein or protein + fat.

*Shake:* This is one that I wouldn't want to try given the PVF choices! But with another PVF choice (like protein powder, spinach, apple, oats, etc.) the shake could be a great option!

*Soup:* Cube the salmon and place in a small pan filled with 2 cups of water. Place the asparagus (chopped in small pieces) and add the avocado oil. Stir in chicken bouillon for flavoring the broth, along with onions, cumin, pepper, oregano, etc. for flavoring. Cook on medium high until the salmon is cooked through and the asparagus is soft.

*Stir-fry:* Cube the salmon and cook in a small pan with the avocado oil on medium heat. In a separate pan, sauté the chopped asparagus in avocado oil, and add any other leftover veggies you have lying around in the fridge. Combine the salmon with the veggies, add sauces, or seasonings, and enjoy!

For this second example, let's go with Ground Turkey (93% lean=P) + Zucchini (V) + Avocado (F).

*Salad:* Brown the ground turkey and season with chili powder, cumin, and sea salt. Throw on top of a bed of leafy greens like spinach and romaine. Dice the zucchini (fresh and raw) and serve diced avocado on top. Add salsa for some delicious moisture and flavor.

*Scramble:* Follow the directions for stir-fry below, but then add liquid egg whites (½ cup) or full eggs (2 eggs=PF) to scramble it up and add extra protein or protein + fat.

*Shake:* This is one that I wouldn't want to try given the PVF choices! But with another PVF choice (like plain Greek yogurt, kale, chia seeds, coconut milk, berries, etc.) the shake could be a great option

*Soup:* Brown the ground turkey and drain the grease. Place the meat in a small pot with 1½ cups water. Dice the zucchini and add to the pot. Season with chicken or beef bouillon, celery salt, oregano, pepper, and thyme, then serve fresh avocado on top of the finished soup.

*Stir-fry:* Brown the turkey in a small pan with the avocado oil on medium heat. When the meat is almost cooked, add in chopped asparagus, as well as any other leftover veggies you have lying around in the fridge. Cook on medium-high until the asparagus and other veggies have softened (add a little water to help cook faster), add a sauce like Primal Kitchen BBQ, sea salt, pepper, and cumin.

Are you starting to get the feel for how you can choose any foods for your PVF or PVFc meal? Once you have selected the foods to use, simply select one of the five S's to figure out a way to easily cook them. This tends to be much easier and more sustainable than trying to make a traditional recipe and tweaking it to fit your goals.

Recipes and gourmet dishes are wonderful to make every now and then, but our quick S-type meals will get the job done day-in and day-out much more quickly. It is so empowering to go about creating a whole new set of meals *you* love using the five S's formula. You will learn which combinations of food you love. Though they're not "traditional," you will soon make them that way in your home because of how good you feel eating them.

## Basic Seasonings, Sauces, and Sweeteners

The "Triple S" as I call it--seasonings, sauces, and sweeteners--are how you can dress up your power foods combinations and make them ultra-tasty! Sometimes, all you will need is sea salt and pepper as the natural flavors of the foods you have chosen are delicious on their own. Other times, you will want to utilize some of your options.

*IMPORTANT:* when you are eating a whole-foods, nutrient-dense diet like the low-carb strategy of the Power Foods Lifestyle, it is important to luxuriously salt your foods to get enough sodium in the day. This may sound counter-

*It is important to luxuriously salt your foods to get enough sodium in the day.*

productive to what society has taught you "healthy" looks like but it is important to do. With a decreased carbohydrate intake, your insulin levels fall significantly, which cause the kidneys to excrete sodium and water in abundance. Sodium is an important electrolyte for regulating the balance of water in and around the cells of your body. If you notice any muscle cramping, water retention, dizziness, or diarrhea, you need to be adding more salt. Use a sea salt or pink Himalayan salt for adding trace minerals to your diet.

I am a big fan of minimalism in the kitchen. Sure, you can go super fancy and make a home-run of a meal every now and then, especially when entertaining, but for sustainability's sake, the normal meal in your life should involve just a few basics.

I have included a list of Triple S products I keep in my kitchen at all times and recommend you start out with as well. You can most definitely add to this list--I just want to get you started in your brainstorming:

| Seasonings | Sauces | Sweeteners |
|---|---|---|
| Sea Salt | Kikkoman Stir-fry Sauce | Stevia (powder) |
| Pepper | Liquid Aminos | Monk Fruit sweetener |
| Oregano | Panda Express Kung Pao | |
| Basil | Heinz BBQ Bold & Spicy | |
| Thyme | Bolthouse Farms yogurt-based dressings (any and all flavors) | |
| Garlic Powder | | |
| Onion Powder | | |
| Chili Powder | | |
| Cumin | | |
| Cinnamon | Primal Kitchen sauces (any and all flavors) | |
| Curry Powder | | |
| Paprika | | |
| Cayenne Pepper | Apple Cider Vinegar | |
| Season-all | Avocado/Olive Oil | |
| Chicken Bouillon | *Any other sauce or dressing that is higher in fat from avocado, olive oil, or avocado oil and low in sugar.* | |
| Beef Bouillon | | |

You can make any combination of food taste wonderful as you explore the Triple S products and get creative. Lean into the discomfort of flavoring your own foods. You just may discover a new taste you never knew you could love!

Let's now move into discussing foods that traditionally use white flours and are higher in carbohydrates. This can include breads, cookies, and other comfort goodies that are common in the Standard American Diet (SAD).

As you explore your new low-carb strategy, you will discover the simple exchange of the flour and sweetener can often bring the carbs down to a level where you can enjoy the food while maintaining your low-carb lifestyle. This may help you decrease any feelings of deprivation you may experience, but I encourage you not to make these types of 'comfort' or 'treat' meals too frequently. Keep these types of food as a fun indulgence only, 1-3x/week or so. Otherwise, it is too easy to stop focusing on the wonderful power foods that should be a standard part of your diet on a regular basis.

Using low-carb flours, like coconut or almond flour, in exchange for white flour is a beneficial practice for shifting the way you cook to be more in line with low-carb. However, it is important to note that these low-carb flours don't generally behave the way that wheat, white, or oat flour does, so you can't just make a 1:1 exchange.

Here are a few quick facts and tips on almond and coconut flour:

Almond Flour:

- » One serving is ¼ cup and contains 6 grams of carbohydrates.
- » It is available in most supermarkets and grocery stores, or can be ordered online.
- » Almond Meal is slightly different than Almond Flour. Almond Meal has the skin of the almonds left on, rather than blanched for removal with flour. While meal is a little coarser, it usually behaves just the same as flour in recipes.
- » Be sure to keep almond flour in an airtight container or in the refrigerator as it can go bad quicker than regular flour.

Coconut Flour:

- » One serving is two Tablespoons and contains 11 grams of carbohydrates.
- » Coconut flour is high in fiber.
- » As discussed above, coconut flour absorbs more liquid than almond flour.
- » Be sure to keep coconut flour in an airtight container away from moisture. One of the best places is on a cool, dark shelf of the pantry.

I hope you enjoy some of the recipes and examples of low-carb alternatives that are in the Sample Meal Plans and Recipes at the end of this book. Just remember to balance those types of meals with our whole-foods, power-type meals and you will be good to go!

> *Remember: low-carb living is about shifting the paradigm in your mind about what constitutes a meal and what does not. You will challenge these old notions on a daily basis and program into your brain what your new normal looks, smells, and tastes like. You will come to love it, especially as you love the way your body feels and functions!*

# Chapter 8:
# Grocery Shopping

Grocery shopping is a critical task when living the low carb strategy of the Power Foods Lifestyle. I have come to enjoy the activity of hand-selecting my foods each week as I shop, and I hope you will too.

I often reflect back on the years that I struggled with my food choices as a high school graduate, college student, and young working professional. Those were often lonely years due to being away from my family, feeling unsure about the direction of my life, sadness over the scoliosis condition that was worsening day by day, and not finding success in dating. During these challenging times, I began shifting away from binging on highly processed, high-carb foods by spending hours in the grocery store aisles on Friday and Saturday evenings. The more I learned about ingredients in foods, the more I found joy in walking the aisles and looking at the ingredient labels in the foods in the store. This activity began to shift my perspective about food, and was a part of the essential shift I made from food as 'coping' to food as 'fuel.' You see, it would be too easy to look at all of the foods I should avoid due to their carbohydrate content and ingredients that cause inflammation in my body and feel sad, as if life isn't fair and my body hates me.

I wonder if you will go through a phase of that too as you decide to say 'good-bye' to many of the foods you formerly ate. But a mindset of scarcity doesn't jive with me, and I hope you will ease yourself into this new mindset as well. Our thoughts determine our emotions, and those emotions then can sway our behavior. As we challenge our thoughts around any activity that feels burdensome, seeking to shift them to a positive light, we find behavior and forming automatic habits that benefit our lives becomes easier. I would like to share three of the aspects of gratitude that have helped me shift my perspective on shopping as I avoid foods that won't help my body function optimally. I am grateful for:

1. the resources to buy my own food,
2. the access to foods brought near my home that I can purchase, and
3. the mobility to get out and buy my own food.

When it comes to enjoying low-carb grocery shopping, I have five simple tips for you:

1. Make your shopping a habit. When it fits your busy lifestyle and time availability, you may utilize the grocery pick-up or even delivery to your home options. This service is becoming more widely available, so if this is something you have access to, and it benefits you, use it! If you prefer to shop "in person", do it! But the more you change it up and alter your schedule or routine, the more you will have difficulty auto-piloting your habits. So, choose a method of how and when you're going to shop and stick with it.

2. As we discussed previously, set an alarm in your phone for the same time each week. This alarm should remind you to sit down and plan your meals so you can make your shopping list and get to the store. Don't just expect yourself to go when it makes sense in your schedule as this adds more anxiety to your life, and less intention to your low-carb lifestyle. It's amazing how many of my one-on-one clients have been blessed by this tip alone! We have so many things going on in our lives, any reminders and gentle nudges in the direction of our goals are helpful.

3. You may already know this, but don't shop hungry. We know the majority of us shop differently when we have a whisper

of hunger in our stomachs. Suddenly, the bakery is the most delightful place on the planet, and we find ourselves fighting down the dragon of rebellion that lurks inside us all. Make sure you've fueled yourself well so you're not tricked by tantalizing smells, colors, and price cuts. Stick to your plan and remind yourself you *love your new lifestyle. (Even if you don't yet--it takes time--so gently remind yourself you're on your way!)*

4. When possible, do a once-a-week shopping trip for the main items you need, then plan a second, smaller produce run for 3-4 days later. Although this can initially feel like overkill, I have found this strategy keeps me loving my low-carb lifestyle as I'm getting fresh, colorful, flavorful produce! That is such a large part of this lifestyle, so do all you can to keep your foods fresh. If this is not an option for you due to lack of time, don't stress it. Keep your produce in the dark cooler (adding a brown paper bag helps, as does wiping off any moisture). Doing this will add a few extra days' life into your veggies. Follow the tips in "Planning Your Meals" as well.

5. Make your list ahead of time (as we discussed in "Planning Your Meals"). Once you know where the majority of your power foods are located, you can structure your list in an efficient manner so you're not wandering the store wasting time. You can get in and out in a strategic manner without backtracking once. When I get to this point with a new store, I feel like it's now my friend! I know where all my stuff is and don't get distracted by foods outside of my normal purchases. You will get there too!

When the season is right, utilize your local Farmer's Markets as well. Locally grown is not only helping the economy, but your food will taste fresher and have more nutrients since it was picked last minute.

# Chapter 9:
# Eating on the Road

Even with a fast-paced lifestyle, you can live a low-carb strategy. Inevitably, you will need to eat some meals while being out and about. You can live a low-carb lifestyle while also prioritizing work, caring for children, and attending outings, parties, and going on vacation.

It is important to train your mind how to think differently according to our meal construction formula and be intentional with your strategies. Additionally, completing my six-week low-carb adaptation challenge is one of the best things you can do to develop automatic habits that will sustain you. I have included more information on this challenge at the end of this book.

One of my favorite sermons ever given was by Elder Dallin H. Oaks entitled "Good, Better, Best." In his teachings, he made it clear that there was a tier from which our behaviors and actions could be derived. There are choices that are good, there are choices that are better, and there are choices that are best.

> *There are choices that are good... choices that are better, and ...choices that are best.*

Within the context of nutrition, there will be times you need to use this teaching to help you select the best option for yourself. The best option will be methodically planning ahead and preparing your own meals for on the go. The better option (a step down from BEST but still awesome) is to look ahead at a menu or call ahead to a host to see what will be available. The good option (a step down from BETTER but still good!) is to simply watch your portions, and mindfully eat with whatever option you have in the moment.

This constant dialogue in your head will serve you as you ask yourself these questions:

*What is a good option?*

*What is my better, or best option?*

*Am I in a space that I can make the best selection for myself?*

No matter which of the good, better, best options you end up with, celebrate the wise choice to fuel your body. Do not take the opportunity to shame yourself. If you know you could have done better, forgive yourself, then simply recalibrate to improve the next time. Think through the various obstacles and decisions you faced that led to your decision and strategize how you can better handle the same decision if faced with it again. This process of retroactive reflection will help improve your approach with each new opportunity.

> *Good Option:* You don't have any say on where you are eating or what foods are being served. But you do have control over the portion size you will eat. You can serve yourself (or order yourself) more protein or fat-based proteins and load up on vegetables, if they're available. You can limit, if not stay away from any sugary dessert options, fruit juices, or other carbs. For example, if you are riding a shuttle to a different state and you stop by a gas station for snacks, you can choose a beef jerky stick, apple, and pack of carrots. You could also choose a hot dog and hold the bun. These aren't BEST choices, but they are still keeping you to a strategy and are good options.

*Better Option:* You know where you will be dining out for a work event and are able to look ahead at the menu online. You strategize ordering a salad with chicken breast and a side of avocado. But when the event arrives, you cave in to peer pressure and eat some of the chips and salsa sitting in the middle of the table, and take a few bites of your friend's dessert. While you have still chosen the better option by having a solid strategic entree, you didn't completely keep refined carbohydrates out. Now, this may be a BEST option for you if you evaluate your psychology, sustainability, and how your body feels. But if this slight indulgence will flare up any pain or health conditions, or even cause a headache later, then this may only have been a Better option for you.

*Best Option:* You know that the restaurant or party you will be going to will not have the best option for your body and for feeling the best you can. So you pack your own food in containers, and prepare simple statements to share with others when they question why you brought your own food: "I have been strategizing my nutrition to experiment with a health condition I've been dealing with" or "I haven't been feeling too well lately so I need to stick to this simple diet I'm on for now—doctor's orders!" It is completely fine to have "little white lies" or even "blame your nutritionist" (ME!) to get people off your back so you can enjoy your low-carb strategy lifestyle.

## Dining Out Options

It would be extremely convenient if we could be told exactly what to eat at any given place we might eat, right? While yes, it would be lovely to be told what to do, it is far more empowering and long-lasting when I teach my clients and you about the principles behind our choices. As you practice implementing these principles, whether at a fast food diner or restaurant, you will quickly find you have the skills to handle any situation with ease.

*Foods to gravitate toward on the menu:*

- Lean protein like chicken breast and turkey*
- Fatty cuts of meat like salmon, pork, bacon, and beef*
- Veggies of all types (butter and oil on them are okay when we hold back on carbs)
- Eggs
- Cheese is fine in smaller amounts
- Avocado
- Salsa, use it instead of a high sugar dressing
- Olives

*If these foods come out in larger portions than you know your body functions best on, ask for a to-go box right away. Cut your meal up and leave only the appropriate portion on your plate to eat. Save the rest in the box underneath your seat for later.

*Foods to gravitate away from:*

- High sugar dressings (Anything over five grams of sugar is considered high sugar)
- Teriyaki or barbeque sauces
- Appetizer options like tortillas, breads, or chips
- Buns, rolls, biscuits, or anything of that nature
- Desserts

These simple principles will become your way of life very soon as you put in the practice. Remember to focus on all that you get to eat instead of all you can't, or better stated, are *choosing* not to eat.

You want your body to feel good, function optimally, and not have any regrets after eating. You choose to fuel and nourish your body, not inflict pain later! You can do this.

# Chapter 10:
# Beverages

Why go to all the work of strategizing your nutrition if you are just going to make up for those dropped carbs by drinking beverages that bring them back in? That would seem counterproductive, right?

Let's get clear on the unoffending beverages you can enjoy and identify those that may trigger flare-ups and pain due to their carbohydrate and/or sugar content.

This section is pretty straight-forward as you look at the chart below. I'll add a few additional thoughts about some of these beverages after you have looked over the sections, noticing the carbohydrate content. Remember: any carbohydrate content over 10 grams is something worth raising your eyebrow at as a future culprit of pain and inflammation. Additionally, the serving size really matters. Most of the beverages below have the macros listed for ONE CUP. One cup is only eight ounces.

*Remember: any carbohydrate content over 10 grams is something worth raising your eyebrows at.*

| SODA POP | | | |
|---|---|---|---|
| Sprite (1 cup) | 0 p | 29 c | 0 f |
| Dr. Pepper (1 cup) | 0 p | 30 c | 0 f |
| MILK | | | |
| 2% Milk (1 cup) | 8 p | 12 c | 5 f |
| Chocolate Milk (1 cup) | 8 p | 26 c | 9 f |
| Unsweetened Almond Milk (1 cup) | 1 p | 1 c | 3 f |
| JUICE | | | |
| Orange Juice (1 cup) | 2 p | 26 c | 1 f |
| Apple Juice (1 cup) | 1 p | 28 c | 0 f |
| Naked Juice (1 cup) | 2 p | 33 c | 0 f |
| "HEALTH" DRINKS | | | |
| Gatorade (1 cup) | 0 p | 14 c | 0 f |
| Kombucha (1 cup) | 0 p | 13 c | 0 f |
| Coconut Water (1 cup) | 0 p | 11 c | 0 f |
| ALCOHOL | | | |
| White Wine (¾ cup) | 0 p | 12 c | 0 f |
| Champagne (¾ cup) | 0 p | 3 c | 0 f |
| Beer (1 cup) | 0 p | 13 c | 0 f |

# Soda Pop

It is clear to see that even eight ounces of your favorite soda pop may not be conducive to a low-carb diet. Naturally, you may wonder if diet soda is a good alternative. As of the writing of this book in 2020, the jury is still out on whether or not artificial sweeteners, which replace the sugar in soda pop, is harmful or not.

Diet drinks are neither "good" nor "bad". It is important to identify if moderate drinking of diet soda contributes to a holistically beneficial, nutrient-dense low-carb diet. If you drink a lot of soda, enough to damage your gut health, then diet soda could be a problem. Some studies have hypothesized that artificial sweeteners cause obesity, which is untrue. While they may be correlated in some measures, it is biochemically impossible to gain fat by consuming any drink with zero calories.

If you consume diet soda, do so moderately. Follow the Power Foods Lifestyle principle of a 1:1 ratio of drinking water for the amount of soda you drink.

## Milk

You may look at this table and see that 2% milk has 12 grams of carbohydrates per cup. *How will I get my calcium if I don't drink milk?* you think. By drinking unsweetened almond or cashew milk, of course! These dairy alternatives have more calcium than average milk. And no, substituting 1% or even skim milk for the 2% doesn't change the carbohydrate amount. This substitution only changes the *fat* amount (we *want* fat grams when following a low-carb strategy!).

Other non-dairy alternatives to milk include unsweetened almond, coconut, flaxseed, walnut, cashew, and hemp milks. If these types of milk are not available at your local grocery store, look at popular health stores like Whole Foods, Sprouts, Good Earth, or online.

## Juice

Isn't it shocking to see the average range of 25-35 grams of carbohydrates per cup of juice? I remember being a senior in high school and realizing I had a lot more energy for my dance classes when I had some apple juice. So naturally, I began filling up my very large water bottles with apple juice to take to dance. For those few weeks, I was probably drinking an average of 4-5 cups of apple juice per day! While the carbs were definitely giving me plenty of energy for my high-intensity activity, I also packed on seven pounds of body fat seemingly overnight. I was very alarmed at this, which was my first realization that *juice was not a health food.*

When you are seeking to keep inflammation out of your body, simply stay away from juice--yes, even if it is fresh-squeezed or 100% natural. Natural sugar, in addition to added sugar, may cause your body to have a flare-up and be in pain. No, it's not fair that we, in chronic pain, have to deal with this--but life rarely is fair. We can do this!

## "Health Drinks"

Gatorade, Kombucha, and Coconut water... isn't it interesting to see how many carbohydrates are in these drinks? Some varieties of Kombucha have a lower amount of carbohydrates, so use wisdom and analysis when finding a drink that may help with your gut health.

There will always be new beverages emerging and marketed as "health drinks". Upon analysis of the macronutrients and ingredients, you can see it for what it really is quickly. You are gaining this awareness and insight to stop being fooled by deceptive words that are exactly what you want to hear.

## Alcohol

While drinking alcohol may slow down weight loss, it isn't completely forbidden in a low-carb diet for those who have a healthy liver. (I hear cheers from those who enjoy a drink here or there!) Choosing the right type of drink, and enjoying it as an infrequent indulgence, is the best way to approach these beverages. Some of the better options include champagne, dry wine, whiskey, and dry martinis.

I hope this chapter helps you think more strategically about what you drink. Whether you can chew it, or simply swallow it, any chemical you ingest will have an impact on your health. If you are shocked at how there really aren't too many options for health-conscious, carb-conscious individuals like you and I, you may wish to adopt one of my philosophies that has served me well.

*I don't drink my calories.*

This means that I will infrequently consume a beverage aside from water. Very rarely are the carbs and sugar worth it. And sometimes, even if there is another "cool product" that emerges, the price is simply not worth it to me! So... I load up my pitcher with chopped cucumbers, lemons, limes, oranges, or even tomatoes and enjoy filling my flask with cold, refreshing water as my main source of life-giving hydration.

I know you will find the right balance for yourself as well.

# Chapter 11:
# Motivation

There is a simple exercise you can do that will make a big difference in your motivation to keep going. Sure, anyone can read this book, listen to a podcast, or talk with a friend or coach and feel motivated! You can get started and feel mountains of momentum from the get-go.

But what happens when you don't have a strategy for how to keep going, and you expect that heightened level of motivation to stay with you? The reality is, it won't. Our human brains don't work this way. What was enticing to us last week or even a few days ago can suddenly not matter today.

That is because we have the same knowledge yet are lacking the emotional strings pulled at that time to facilitate the same energy. Therefore, we must have a way to pull our emotional strings down the road to keep the energy present and desire to keep going strong. Yes, ultimately this should and will become a lifestyle full of automaticity. However, habits and automaticity are earned as the reward for diligent, persistent actions that slowly get etched deeper into the brain.

Whenever I speak with my clients, the topic of the driving force for their efforts comes up. All too often, we are driven to improve our eating due to a fear of what others think about our physical appearance, fear of becoming ill, or shame of not measuring up to a standard we feel like we should be meeting. Each of these negative drivers may get us started but won't last long in carrying us through the journey. Over time, these drivers wear and tear us down so our self-esteem erodes in the process of improving our health, pain, and energy.

How different an experience it is when an individual can navigate to the place within themselves where they take ownership of their actions. They desire to improve, and to be a little better than they were the day before. The individual who seeks to motivate from a place of calm, love, and opportunity will always achieve more than the individual who motivates from a place of fear and shame. The best way you can achieve this is to daily take a quick moment to review why you are seeking to make these changes.

Spiritually speaking, when your spirit practices the agency to temper and discipline the body, for which the spirit craved adjoining, there is a spiritual frequency achieved. This brings a state of happiness and enlightenment and is often missed entirely by seekers of health who are solely focused on the status of the body. When the spirit and the body are combined and the individual uses spiritual discipline and a desire to be the master of him or herself, greater power can be found within.

I have made a list below of some of the most frequently-arising statements of motivation that my clients and I have used. Write down the phrases that resonate with you on a 3x5" card. This card should be placed somewhere you will see it often, bringing frequently to mind the reason you are focusing on pulling away from carbs as a fuel source, and gravitating toward proteins, vegetables, and fats.

I am fueling my body strategically so that I can:

» Have more sustainable energy throughout the day.

» Feel more vibrant in my body.

» Feel more alert in my mind.

» Reduce the achiness in my joints.

» Stop my body from flaring up in pain.

» Feel more confident in the way I look.

» Get rid of the bloat I seem to always carry around.

- » Feel more at peace within my spirit for how I am caring for this body.
- » Improve my integrity with myself and follow through on what I say I'm going to do.

You have the power to take your nutrition into your own hands.

There is a lot of noise out there in our world about how you should be eating to reach certain goals.

No doubt you will continue to hear information, some of it useful, and some not so much.

Use the methodology and principles you have learned in this book as a foundation you can return to again and again.

You will continue to evolve as you learn new information, or gain perspective on information you already have attained. You can bring in those "frames" to work with your foundation in a manner you decide.

But I urge you to keep this foundation. It will help you feel grounded, calm, and assured as you face the whirlwinds of "advice" available out there in what I call "the abyss" of social media, blogosphere, podcasts, and books.

Now, lest you suddenly start calling non-strategic carbs 'bad,' let's discuss this. When it comes to a sustainable lifestyle with a healthy psychology, it is important to have constructive dialogue in our heads. That is one reason I call these carbs non-strategic rather than 'bad.' Can you have them? Sure! Does that make you a bad person? No! Might your body experience some symptoms of inflammation, pain, raised blood sugar, and/or headaches if you eat non-strategic carbs? Perhaps!

At the end of the day, you get to proactively choose this lifestyle and adhere to the recommendations made in this book. That personal ownership over your choices is everything and will turn a "rebellion-oriented tendency" into a "compliance-oriented tendency." Trust in yourself. Believe in yourself. Be mindful of the words you use around foods. Yes, other people will continue to use their verbiage programmed by society's ideals. Don't seek to correct them, simply use your new lingo when you have the chance to speak. This usually opens up the opportunity to share what you have learned with others and influence them to approach a healthier relationship with food.

When you can define what eating non-strategically, or even too many power carbs, is doing to your body, you can better find the underlying motivation for why you will focus on fueling your body with PVF meals instead. For the sake of this example, I will use the term "carbs" to encompass both non-strategic as well as too many power carbs:

> *Pain:* Is eating carbs causing your body to be inflamed? Do you notice an extra achiness in your joints, and sensitivity in your muscles? Do carbs bring about headaches--whether tension, migraine, or cluster?
>
> *Lack of Confidence:* Is eating carbs part of what is holding you overweight, or above a weight that helps you feel confident not only in how you look, but how you move and the activities in which you can participate? Are carbs associated with how you cope with life circumstances that feel out of your control, and are part of what holds you hostage to a less-than-stellar outlook on life due to how they make your body feel?
>
> *Health Conditions:* Is eating carbs leading to a heightened blood sugar that puts you at risk for Type 2 Diabetes? Is eating carbs contributing to a build-up of plaque in your arteries, putting you at risk for heart disease? Is eating carbs contributing to inflammation and other symptoms for another health condition you are experiencing?
>
> Digestion: Is eating carbs causing your bowel movements to be either loose, frequent, and unpredictable? Or perhaps you notice that bowel movements are less frequent due to your intake of carbs? Is eating carbs making you gassy, especially the

fierce-smelling ones that can be quite embarrassing? Is eating carbs causing your gut to bloat, look distended, and hold water throughout your body?

The last thing I want you to walk away from this instructional book thinking is, *"Gosh, she really hates carbs and doesn't want anyone to ever enjoy life again by eating non-strategic carbs!"*

That isn't the case at all. I want to see you empower yourself to take ownership, and better understand how these types of carbohydrates impact you.

Nutrition is so extremely nuanced that it gets trickier and trickier to teach on a large scale. Working one-on-one is a far more productive way to ensure the individual gets exactly what they need as we figure their body out. But I also know the methods I teach in this book work on a large scale *if you will apply the principle of listening to your body and experimenting on the method.*

» Three months from now, you may find you do best on a true PVF lifestyle with no carbs.

» Three months from now, you may find you do best on a PVF lifestyle with a power carb after workouts.

» Three months from now, you may find you do best on a PVF lifestyle with a non-strategic carb every few days because you find joy in it, and it's worth whatever symptoms you experience to have that little food "delight".

» Three months from now, you may find your body is actually capable of having a PVC or a PVF meal fluidly throughout the day, and that your body responds well to both energy sources of Carbs and Fats so long as you keep to 80%+ power foods and watch your portion sizes.

The end goal will look different for all of us! And that speaks volumes about just how unique we all are. While principles of nutrition are helpful and give us structure, the overarching principles of agency and ownership shine brightly, taking us to the next level of functioning.

Let me backup just a moment though, as the phrase "end goal" isn't right. You see, there is no "end goal". There is no finish line... that is, until we pass from this life and are no longer in need of nourishing this physical vehicle for the spirit.

So instead of striving for some indeterminable level of sustainability, *strive instead to feel good in your body, take ownership of your choices, and love your life today.* This goal should be written in a dry erase marker on your bathroom mirror so you remember it and have it in the forefront of your mind every day. When you focus on today, you live more fully. You do not put off happiness for some future that never arrives. All you have is today. As you practice reaching a wonderful today, your tomorrow that becomes your today will look different. In contrast, today becomes simpler, where you experience fewer symptoms and physical distress than before.

Isn't that wonderful? That is a goal worth striving for.

Say it out loud with me three times:

# I will strive to feel good in my body, take ownership of my choices, and love my life today.

Today is a new day, and a new opportunity for you to feel better inside and out.

Food is fuel.

Be intentional with your eating.

It's not about the food.

But the food certainly has an impact on our lives.

From this day forward, you will now use food strategically to fuel your vehicle.

You can do it!

Take it one meal, one workout, and one day at a time.

# Chapter 12:
# Sample Meal Plans

These sample meal plans are designed for adult women. Caloric needs differ from person to person, so the portions and numbers provided are based on averages as seen in my coaching practice. Women ages 65+ generally need calories to be around 1,500-1,600 for maintenance while active women generally need calories to be around 2,200-2,500 for maintenance.

The plans below are a great starting point, with calories designed for the average female maintenance weight of 1,700-2,000 calories. I have designed them to be the most average meal intake of three main meals per day with a mid-afternoon and evening snack. You can combine meals together if you desire to eat fewer meals per day, or even do Intermittent Fasting style where you eat your PVF-based meals all in a narrow time window of 4-8 hours per day.

If you notice yourself losing weight but don't want to, simply increase the portion sizes of a few meals to bring the calories up by a few hundred. Alternatively, if you notice yourself feeling better but not losing weight (and you want to), reduce the portion sizes of a few meals slightly to bring the calories down by a few hundred. Weight loss, maintenance, and gain are all dependent on total calorie intake. So, you can eat low-carb and enjoy the benefits no matter which of those three body composition categories you are in.

## Protein Powder

Some of the meals in the sample meal plans include protein powder. This is a convenient way to help your body get the amount of protein it needs in a day to meet this low-carb strategy criteria, especially when minding the principles of the Power Foods Lifestyle like:

» Only eat meat 1-3x/day

» Only eat red meat 1-3x/week

When you observe those principles, you can get enough protein in the day if you eat eggs and a dairy form of protein (like cottage cheese or Greek yogurt). But in the case of many of my clients, they either have a dislike for, or allergy to, eggs or dairy products. This leaves a gap in the necessary protein which we need to fill with protein powder.

Yes, there is some protein in complex carbs like beans and legumes, but we are trying to reduce those power foods in your diet. Yes, there is some great protein in power fats like nuts and seeds, but once you start getting more than ½ cup in your day, anecdotal evidence and experience shows constipation begins to occur.

The protein powder in these meals can be any bone broth powder, whey, egg, or vegan powder. View some of my recommendations below:

*Bone Broth:* Sun, Cow, Grass (unflavored--add your own flavoring using vanilla extract, almond extract, baking cocoa, or most of the blended shakes in these menus will taste great without a flavored protein)

*Whey:* Dymatize (brownie) or Clean Simple Eats (vanilla cake)

*Egg:* Jay Robb (vanilla)

*Plant-Based:* Organi Organic Protein (creamy chocolate) or Sunwarrior Protein Warrior Blend (chocolate)

Customized portions for caloric needs are often helpful for those who simply don't have time to calculate it all, or experience anxiety over not knowing if what you're doing is right for you. Please visit www.PowerFoodsLifestyle.com/coaching to learn how to work with me on a one-on-one level for customization, accountability, and adaptation to life circumstances.

Customizing your own plan can feel intimidating, in spite of knowing the science and information of *what* to do. So, if implementation is something you know you could use some oomph in, please reach out for coaching. It's an investment in yourself worth making. In addition to finding the right plan, there is something to be said for the power of accountability.

The American Society of Training and Development (ASTD) conducted a study which found an individual is 65% more likely to complete a goal when they commit to someone not within their normal circle of influence. But that percentage of achievement jumps up to 95% when setting a specific accountability appointment with the person to whom you have committed. So, if working with me isn't an option, go out of your way to recruit another mentor or friend who can take on that accountability responsibility for you. Set up regular appointments and check-ins, whether through phone calls, emails, text messages, or video chat. Track your progress, your efforts, and your outcomes so you can measure what you are doing that is working or isn't working, and make tweaks from there (all of these trackers are built into my 6-week Low-Carb Challenge).

*"When performance is measured, performance improves. When performance is measured and reported, the rate of improvement accelerates."* — *Thomas S. Monson*

| SAMPLE MEAL PLAN GUIDE TO MACRO ACRONYMS |
| --- |
| *As you observe the sample meal plans, you can assess portion size using the following acronym and their macronutrient "peak ranges" set forth by the Power Foods Lifestyle.* |
| Key for Power Foods Lifestyle Acronyms and Macros: |
| P = 15-30 grams protein |
| p = 7.5-15 grams protein |
| V = ½-2 cups vegetables |
| F = 8-12 grams fat |
| f = 4-6 grams fat |
| C = 20-30 grams carbohydrates |
| c = 10-15 grams carbohydrates |

# Meal Plan 1

Breakfast: (Scrambled Chicken Eggs with Avocado on Top)

    (pf) 1 whole egg
    (p) 2 oz. chopped chicken
    (V) 1 c. broccoli (chopped small)
    (F) 2 oz. avocado

Lunch: (Salad)

    (P) 4 oz. chicken breast (cubed)
    (V) 2 handfuls leafy greens
    (V) ½ Roma tomato (diced)
    (c) ½ medium apple
    (F) 12 raw almonds
    (F) 2 tsp. Avocado oil

Snack: (Stir)

    (P) ⅔ c. plain Greek yogurt
    (V) 2 stalks celery
    (F) 1 Tbsp. almond or peanut butter (natural)

Dinner: (Grilled Patty with Steamed Vegetables)

    (PF) 4 oz. grass-fed beef patty-85% lean
    (V) 1 c. steamed cauliflower
    (V) 1 c. steamed green beans
    (c) 2 oz. steamed sweet potato
    (F) 2 tsp. extra virgin olive oil

Bedtime Snack: (Warm Protein Drink)

    (P) 1 serving protein powder
    (V) ½ c. sliced cucumber
    (f) 1 c. unsweetened almond milk + ½ c. water
    (f) 1 tsp. Coconut oil

# Meal Plan 2

Breakfast: (Cottage Cheese Parfait)

    (P) ½ c. cottage cheese (2%) with cinnamon
    (V) 1 c. sugar snap peas - (eat on the side)
    (F) 2 Tbsp. chopped walnuts
    (c) ¼ c. chopped raspberries

Lunch: (Soup--quadruple and make 4 days' worth in bulk)

    (P) 4 oz. turkey breast
    (V) ½ c. green beans (canned or fresh)
    (V) ½ c. zucchini (diced)
    (V) ½ c. orange or red bell pepper (diced)
    (V) 1 c. collard greens (chopped)
    (F) 1 tsp. extra virgin olive oil

Snack: (Diced Eggs)

    (PF) 2 hard-boiled eggs (consider adding a little mustard for flavor)
    (V) 1/2 c. cucumber (diced)

Dinner: (Stir-fry)

    (P) 4 oz. chicken breast (cubed)
    (V) 1 c. kale (chopped)
    (V) ½ c. summer squash (diced)
    (V) ½ c. asparagus
    (F) 1 Tbsp. grass-fed butter or ghee
    (c) 2 small red potatoes (70 grams-diced)

Bedtime Snack: (Chocolate Peanut Butter Bark)

    (F) 2 tsp. coconut oil
    (F) 1 Tbsp. natural peanut butter
    » Mix in a ½ tsp. cocoa powder with a dash of stevia. Mix well and freeze until solid.

# Meal Plan 3

Breakfast: (Sausage Scramble)

    (P) 3 oz. natural chicken sausage
    (pf) 1 whole egg
    (V) 1 c. collard greens
    (V) 1 c. diced bell pepper and onions
    (F) 2 tsp. avocado oil

Lunch: (Shake)

    (P) 1 serving protein powder
    (V) 1 c. spinach
    (V) 1 stalk celery
    (F) 1 Tbsp. natural peanut butter
    (f) 2 tsp. Chia seeds
    (f) 1 c. unsweetened almond milk + ½-1 cup water
    (c) ½ c. mixed berries

Snack: (Lettuce Wraps)

    (P) 3 oz. deli turkey breast (nitrate-free)
    (V) 3 leaves green leaf lettuce
    (F) ½ c. black olives

Dinner: (Salad)

    (P) 4 oz. chicken breast (cubed)
    (V) 2 c. mixed spring greens
    (V) ½ c. broccoli (chopped)
    (V) ½ c. cauliflower (chopped)
    (V) ½ Roma tomato (diced)
    (F) 2 Tbsp. pumpkin seeds
    (pF) 2 strips bacon (natural--chopped)

Bedtime Snack: (No-Bake Cookie Ball)

    (c) 2 Tbsp. rolled oats
    (F) 1 Tbsp. natural peanut butter
    (-) 2 tsp. Swerve (low-carb low sugar powdered sugar)

# Meal Plan 4

Breakfast: (Over-Easy Eggs over Veggies)

    (PF) 2 whole eggs
    (V) 1 c. steamed zucchini
    (V) 1 c. steamed summer squash

Lunch: (Stir-fry)

    (P) 4 oz. lean pork
    (V) 1 c. brussels sprouts (sliced)
    (V) ½ c. carrots (sliced)
    (F) 2 tsp. extra virgin olive oil
    (F) 2 oz. avocado

Snack: (Shake)

    (P) 1 serving protein powder (in 10-12 oz. water)
    (V) ½ c. jicama (sliced--eat on the side)
    (F) 2 Tbsp. raw pecans (eat on the side)

Dinner: (Oven Bake)

    (PF) 4 oz. salmon (cubed)
    (V) ½ c. cauliflower
    (V) ½ c. asparagus (cut in 2" lengths)
    (V) ½ c. red bell pepper
    (F) 2 tsp. avocado oil (brushed on top before baking)

Bedtime Snack: (Cottage Cheese Snack)

    (P) ½ c. cottage cheese (2%) mixed with cinnamon and a little stevia sweetener
    (V) ½ c. sugar snap peas (on the side)
    (F) 12 raw almonds

# Meal Plan 5

Breakfast: (Blueberry Crepes)

    (P) 4 large egg whites
    (F) 3 Tbsp. almond flour (mix with egg whites and a little water)
    (c) ½ c. blueberries (add stevia for a little sweetener)

Lunch: (Salad)

    (P) 4 oz. tuna
    (pf) 1 hard-boiled egg
    (V) 1 c. spring lettuce mix
    (V) 1 c. chopped purple cabbage
    (F) 2 oz. avocado
    (f) 2 tbsp. Bolthouse Farms ranch dressing

Snack: (Grab-n-Go)

    (PF) 2 Nick's Sticks beef sticks
    (V) 5 baby carrots
    (F) 2 Brazil nuts

Dinner: (Kabobs)

    (P) 4 oz. chicken breast (cubed)
    (V) ¼ bell pepper (diced)
    (V) ½ c. zucchini (diced)
    (V) ½ c. summer squash (diced)
    (c) 2 oz. sweet potato (cubed)
    (F) 2 tsp. avocado oil (brushed on top before baking)
    (F) 2 oz. avocado (serve with cooked kabobs)

Bedtime Snack: (Shake)

    (P) 1 serving protein powder
    (V) ½ c. sugar snap peas (on the side)
    (F) 12 raw almonds

# COMPLETE THE 6-WEEK LOW-CARB LIFESTYLE CHALLENGE

If you liked those sample meal plans and recipes, you will love my 6-week Challenge program. I designed this program to help you have a solid plan to follow as you learn these principles of low-carb living, and have a methodical way to test at which level of carb intake you feel best.

While I wrote this challenge primarily for women, the adaptation for adding calories for men is simple and explained in the challenge. So, ladies, if your husband or partner wants to give this a try, it will be perfect for him also.

The Challenge Includes:

- » 6 Menus to follow (1 per week)
    - o Simple Meal Preparation Suggestions
- » Suggestions for Meal Timing
    - o 3 meals/day, 4 meals/day, and 5 meals/day (choose your style)
- » 10 Family Dinner Recipes
    - o They have a Low-Carb base and suggestions on how to incorporate carbs for the rest of the family, if desired
- » Grocery Shopping List (1 per week)
    - o Written for one person, but can be adapted for a full family
- » 6 Low-Carb Dessert Recipes (1 per week)
    - o A great way to enjoy something sweet without losing strategy
- » Complete Food Exchange List
    - o For variety and ideas to change things up
- » Accountability and Habits Tracker

- o Includes space for a weekly journal entry to assess how you are feeling and the low-carb lifestyle feels in your body
» Approved Sauces, Seasonings, and Sweeteners
- o Get all the right products in your kitchen
» Weight and Measurements Tracker
- o You only need to use this if losing weight is a goal along with reducing inflammation in your body
» Protein Powder & Supplement Recommendations
- o I am not tied to any particular company, so recommend what works from multiple companies!

*Get Your Copy of the Challenge and low-carb Recipe Book at*
*www.PowerFoodsLifestyle.com*

# Sample Recipes

For more tasty recipes, please visit:
www.PowerFoodsLifestyle.com

# Sunrise Stir-fry

18p / 8c / 16f / 233cal

*Recipe Yield: 1 serving*

Ingredients

| | |
|---|---|
| 2 large egg whites | 2 tsp. coconut oil |
| ¾ c. frozen stir-fry vegetables | 2 tsp. sea salt |
| ⅛ c. water | ⅛ tsp. pepper |
| 1 strip bacon | ¼ tsp. chili powder |

*Directions*

1. Use kitchen scissors to cut the bacon in small pieces. Cook the bacon on medium-high heat in a medium skillet.
2. Remove the bacon from the pan. Pour the vegetables into the bacon grease with an additional ⅛ cup of water. Cook on high, stirring occasionally, until vegetables are a light golden brown.
3. Add the coconut oil to the skillet and continue stirring. Reduce heat to medium-high.
4. Crack in the eggs and add the bacon pieces back in. Scramble all together.
5. Mix in the seasonings and continue scrambling until eggs are cooked to desired doneness.

*Additional Notes*

» One sausage link can replace the bacon strip.
» Use only egg whites if you wish to have diced avocado on top without adding additional calories.
» Change up the type of veggies used in this dish to enjoy some variety.

# Weightless Waffles

24p / 10c / 8f / 220cal

*Recipe Yield: 7 servings*

*Ingredients*

    24 large egg whites (3 cups liquid egg whites)
    ½ c. unsweetened almond milk
    3 servings vanilla protein powder (90 grams)
    2 tsp. Baking powder
    ½ c. almond flour
    ⅔ c. coconut flour

*Directions*

1. Combine egg whites, protein powder, and baking powder in a large mixing bowl. Whip until well mixed.
2. Stir in the almond meal and coconut flour until mixed thoroughly.
3. Add in almond milk to achieve the texture of pancake batter. Mix well.
4. Spray waffle iron with a non-stick oil. Pour ¾ c. batter into the center of the griddle.

*Additional Notes*

» These waffles can be made in bulk and frozen in a Ziplock bag. Reheat on a cookie sheet in the oven or cut apart to toast.

» Try topping with a light spread of natural peanut or almond butter, unsweetened coconut flakes, and sliced almonds. Sprinkle with stevia powder for sweetener.

# Egg and Turkey Bites

29p / 4c / 12f / 240cal

*Recipe Yield: 7 servings*

*Ingredients*

> ½ lb. ground turkey breast (90% lean)
> 28 large eggs (or 14 large eggs and 1 ⅔ c. liquid egg whites)
> 1 bell pepper (any color)
> chili powder
> sea salt

*Directions*

1. Brown the ground turkey in a large skillet on medium-high heat. Drain the grease.
2. Use a non-stick cooking spray to generously coat 14 muffin tin cups.
3. Spoon the cooked ground turkey into each cup. Distribute evenly between the 14 cups.
4. Wash the bell pepper. Dice into very small pieces after cutting off the stem and removing the seeds. Distribute the diced pepper between the 14 cups.
5. Crack one whole egg into each tin. Scramble the yolk with a fork. Add an additional egg white or 3 Tbsp. liquid egg white to each tin until the egg is nearly at the level of the flat part of the tin.
6. Lightly sprinkle the chili powder and sea salt on top of each egg in the tin.
7. Bake at 400 degrees Fahrenheit for 20-25 minutes or until eggs are lightly browned and firm to the touch.

*Additional Notes*

» These eggs can be made in bulk and stored in the refrigerator for up to 4 days. Reheat in the microwave for 30 seconds per muffin.

» Experiment by adding different vegetables like grated zucchini, carrots, or chopped spinach.

# Eat Olive It

16p / 8c / 8.5f / 205cal

*Recipe Yield: 1 serving*

*Ingredients*

> ½ c. cottage cheese (2%)
> 5 med. baby carrots
> 1 stalk celery
> 10 large olives (any variety)
> 1 tsp. ranch powder mix

*Directions*

1. Wash the celery thoroughly.
2. Place cottage cheese in a bowl and stir in ranch powder mix.
3. Dice the carrots and celery.
4. Slice the olives into thirds.
5. Drop diced vegetables and cut olives into cottage cheese.

*Additional Notes*

» Substitute a palmful of raw almonds, walnuts, macadamia nuts, or pumpkin seeds for the olives, or do a ½ and ½ portion to experience a variety of textures and flavors.

# Mashed Tuna and Veggies

30p / 9c / 10f / 290cal

*Recipe Yield: 1 serving*

*Ingredients*

>1 can tuna - 4 oz. (packed in water)
>½ medium avocado
>2 celery stalks
>1 tsp. Dijon mustard
>⅛ tsp. pepper

*Directions*

1. Drain the tuna.
2. Scoop the avocado into a bowl.
3. Mash the tuna into the avocado with a fork.
4. Mix in the mustard and pepper and mash together well.
5. Use the celery stalks to scoop up the tuna and avocado mixture.

*Additional Notes*

» Try using different vegetables to dip in the tuna (like broccoli florets) or dice them and mix in (like a bell pepper, sliced carrots, or diced onions).

# Yolks and Sprouts

27p / 5c / 9f / 234cal

*Recipe Yield: 1 serving*

Ingredients

>    3 med. Brussels sprouts
>    2 large eggs
>    ½ c. liquid egg whites (4 large egg whites)
>    sea salt (to taste)
>    pepper (to taste)
>    ¼ tsp. garlic powder

*Directions*

1. Wash the Brussels sprouts. Cut off the stem, then slice each sprout into thin slices.
2. Place the sliced sprouts in a small skillet. Add enough water to cover the bottom of the pan.
3. Cook the sprouts on medium high, stirring often, and adding a little water as needed to keep from scalding. Season with garlic powder, sea salt, and pepper.
4. Remove sprouts from the pan. Spray the pan with a non-stick cooking oil. Reduce heat to medium, then crack in the eggs.
5. Allow to cook until the egg white has turned from clear to white. Flip over, keeping the yolk intact to make over-easy eggs.
6. Once the eggs have finished cooking, add on top of the sprouts.
7. Spray the pan once more with non-stick cooking oil. Scramble the egg whites on medium heat. Season with sea salt and pepper.
8. Serve scrambled whites over the over-easy eggs and cooked sprouts, letting the yolk run over the entire dish.

*Additional Notes*

- » If in a hurry, simply scramble the egg whites and whole eggs together. However, the runny yolk is delightful enough to warrant a few extra minutes!
- » The Brussels sprouts could be substituted with cauliflower, broccoli, or even bok choy.

# Honey Ginger Kabobs

28p / 18c / 13f / 325cal

*Recipe Yield: 4 servings*

*Ingredients*

    1 lb. chicken breast
    2 bell peppers (any color)
    1 medium summer squash
    1 medium zucchini
    ¼ yellow onion

    <u>Marinade</u>
    ⅓ c. extra virgin olive oil
    ⅓ c. tomato sauce
    1 Tbsp. raw honey
    3 Tbsp. liquid aminos
    1 Tbsp. ginger
    2 tsp. paprika

*Directions*

1. Wash, trim the fat, and cube the chicken breast into 1" chunks.
2. Wash the bell pepper, squash, and zucchini. Remove the stem and seeds from the bell pepper before cutting into 1" wide chunks.
3. Slice the zucchini and summer squash lengthwise to make large chunks.
4. Cube the onion.
5. Coat the skewers with a little non-stick cooking spray to prevent them from burning.
6. Alternately skewer the chicken, squash, zucchini, bell pepper, and onion. Arrange the colors to be high contrasting.
7. Place skewers side-by-side in a storage container that has a lid.
8. Mix the marinade together in a small mixing bowl. Pour

marinade over chicken skewers. Cover with the lid and refrigerate for at least 4 hours.

9. Grill kabobs on the barbeque or bake in the oven at 325 degrees Fahrenheit for 30-35 minutes or until chicken is cooked all the way through.

*Additional Notes*

» For more variety: Swap out chicken for pork, salmon, or hamburger.

» For a slightly higher carbohydrate count, add cubed sweet potato to the mix.

# Lemon Cilantro Fish

24p / 8c / 10f / 275cal

*Recipe Yield: 4 servings*

*Ingredients*

    1 lb. fish filets (tilapia, tuna - cut into 4-oz. filets)
    4 c. spinach leaves
    4 c. arugula
    2 Roma tomatoes
    2 medium avocados

    <u>Marinade</u>
    ¼ c. extra virgin olive oil
    ¼ c. unsweetened almond milk
    3 Tbsp. lemon juice
    1 Tbsp. cilantro
    1 Tbsp. paprika
    1 Tbsp. garlic salt
    1 tsp. parsley
    1 tsp. sea salt
    1 tsp. Red pepper flakes (optional for more heat)

*Directions*

1. In a medium mixing bowl, combine the marinade ingredients. Mix well.
2. Wash the fish filets, then place in a storage container that has a lid. Pour marinade over the filets. Cover with a lid and refrigerate for 3-4 hours.
3. Bake filets at 375 degrees Fahrenheit for 30 minutes, or until the fish easily flakes apart.
4. Rinse and chop the leafy greens along with the tomato.
5. Serve a 4-oz. filet with ½ diced tomato over 1 c. spinach and 1 c. arugula. Dice half an avocado and add to the salad.

*Additional Notes*

- » Salmon can be used for this meal, though the fat amount will be increased by 12 grams which is about 110 calories.
- » A light balsamic dressing or avocado oil can be drizzled on top with a few more fat grams and calories. To keep lighter on calories, use fresh lemon juice or salsa.
- » Experiment with different types of leafy greens: chard, kale, romaine, or collard greens.

# Juicy Chicken Bites and Guac

31p / 11c / 13f / 350cal

*Recipe Yield: 4 servings*

*Ingredients*

    1 lb. chicken breast
    2 medium zucchinis
    2 tsp. avocado oil

    *Marinade*
    3 Tbsp. apple cider vinegar
    3 Tbsp. extra virgin olive oil
    ½ tsp. paprika
    chicken rub or seasoning of your choice
    sea salt (to taste)

    *Guac*
    1 medium avocado
    ½ c. cottage cheese (2%)
    1 Tbsp. unsweetened almond milk
    1 Tbsp. ranch powder mix
    1 tsp. chili powder
    sea salt and pepper (to taste)

*Directions*

1. Wash and trim the fat off the chicken breast. Cut chicken into bite-sized cubes.
2. Combine the apple cider vinegar, olive oil, paprika, salt, and chicken rub in a bowl. Mix well.
3. Place the cubed chicken in a storage container with a lid. Pour the marinade over the chicken and place the lid on top. Refrigerate for 4 hours.
4. Preheat the oven to 350 degrees Fahrenheit.
5. Wash the zucchini. Slice in ¼" thick rounds. Toss in a hot skillet on medium heat with a very small amount of avocado oil until the edges are browned. Sprinkle with sea salt.

6. In a small bowl, combine avocado, cottage cheese, and almond milk with a hand blender. Once the mixture is smooth, stir in the remaining seasonings. Add a few dashes of sea salt and pepper.
7. Place chicken in a glass dish or on a cookie sheet lined with tin foil for easy clean-up. Bake for 30-35 minutes or until meat is cooked all the way through.
8. Serve chicken and zucchini with avocado dip on the side.

*Additional Notes*

» Change up the vegetable or add more to enjoy more color. Try sliced Brussels sprouts, diced bell pepper, thin carrot sticks, or cauliflower florets.

# Lemon Pepper Squash Salad

39p / 20c / 13f / 375cal

*Recipe Yield: 1 serving*

*Ingredients*

    1 c. romaine lettuce
    1 c. spinach leaves
    4 oz. lean ground beef (90%+ lean)
    ½ c. summer squash (diced)
    2 mini sweet peppers
    ¼ c. diced onion
    ½ Roma tomato
    1 lemon
    sea salt (to taste)
    ½ Tbsp. oregano
    pepper (to taste)

*Directions*

1. Brown the hamburger in a skillet. Drain the grease. Liberally sprinkle with sea salt and oregano.
2. Wash the leafy greens, summer squash, peppers, and tomato.
3. Dice the summer squash, tomato, onion, and peppers. Chop the leafy greens.
4. This salad can be eaten with raw vegetables. For softer vegetables:
   - Place the peppers, squash, and onions in a small skillet with ⅓ c. water. Cook on medium-high or until the water is gone. Stir regularly.
   - Cook for a few minutes longer on medium heat to get the edges of the vegetables crispy.
   - Pile the meat, vegetables, and tomato on top of the leafy greens.
   - Cut the lemon in half and squeeze onto the salad for moisture and flavor.
   - Sprinkle lightly with pepper.

*Additional Notes*

- » If using a leaner meat like ground turkey or chicken breast, add additional fats like diced avocado, avocado oil as a dressing, and/or pumpkin seeds.
- » For additional calories and fat grams, add 1 Tbsp. sunflower seeds, 1 Tbsp. pumpkin seeds, and use a fat-based dressing like Tessemae's or Primal Kitchen.

# Chocolate Fudge Bombs

3p / 6c / 12f / 160cal

*Recipe Yield: 16 servings*

*Ingredients*

- 4 Tbsp. coconut oil
- 4 Tbsp. dark baking cocoa
- ¾ c. almond flour
- ⅔ c. peanut butter
- ¼ c. unsweetened almond milk
- 2 Tbsp. honey *(or substitute 1 Tbsp. stevia for even fewer carbs)*
- 2 tsp. cinnamon

*Directions*

1. Heat coconut oil until liquid. Mix in baking cocoa and almond flour.
2. In a separate bowl, mix slightly heated peanut butter with almond milk, honey, and cinnamon.
3. Mix both bowls together.
4. Spread batter in a square pan that has been lightly sprayed with non-stick oil.
5. Cover with tin foil and freeze for 20 minutes until set before serving.
6. Cut 4x4 rows for 16 small squares before serving. Do not leave outside the freezer for too long or they will melt.

*Additional Notes*

» Try substituting almond butter for peanut butter.

» Add a little almond meal for firmer fudge squares.

» Layer unsweetened coconut flakes, chopped walnuts, or slivered almonds on top for more texture and crunch without too many more carbs.

# Chocolate Blueberry Pudding

13p / 17c / 11f / 215cal

*Recipe Yield: 1 serving*

*Ingredients*

> ½ c. plain Greek yogurt (2%)
> ⅓ c. blueberries
> 2 tsp. dark baking cocoa
> 1 Tbsp. peanut butter
> ½ tsp. stevia powder

*Directions*

> Wash the blueberries and combine with yogurt in a small mixing bowl.
>
> Use a hand blender to puree the blueberries into the yogurt.
>
> Mix in the remaining ingredients.

*Additional Notes*

» Reduce the carbs further by cutting out the blueberries.

» Experiment with different types of berries for a variety of flavor.

» Swap out cottage cheese for yogurt, if desired.

# Chocolate Candy Bar Shake

29p / 12c / 13f / 290cal

*Recipe Yield: 1 serving*

*Ingredients*

> 1 c. unsweetened almond milk
> ½ c. warm water
> 1 serving chocolate protein powder (30 g)
> or add 2 tsp. dark baking cocoa to a vanilla protein
> 1 Tbsp. peanut butter
> ¼ tsp. stevia powder
> ⅛ tsp. almond extract

*Directions*

1. Combine all ingredients in a shaker bottle or blender. Mix thoroughly.
2. Though this shake can be made with cold water, serve warm for a satisfying experience, particularly in the evening or in colder weather.

*Additional Notes*

» Try substituting almond or cashew butter for peanut butter.

» If using a blender, mix in a handful of spinach or kale for additional nourishment to make a full PVF meal.

# Peanut Butter Brownie Cake

24p / 14c / 7f / 220cal

*Recipe Yield: 3 servings*

## Ingredients

- 5 large egg whites (¾ cup liquid egg whites)
- 2 servings chocolate protein powder (60 g)
- ⅓ c. unsweetened almond milk
- ½ tsp. vanilla extract
- 1 tsp. cinnamon
- 2 Tbsp. natural peanut butter
- 1 Tbsp. honey (or ½ Tbsp. stevia powder)

## Directions

1. Whip the egg whites, protein powder, and milk (add almond milk slowly).
2. Stir in the honey, vanilla, and cinnamon. Final texture should be like cake batter.
3. Pour batter into a square baking dish lightly greased with non-stick cooking spray.
4. Bake at 350 degrees Fahrenheit for 8-12 minutes or until brownies are firm to the touch.
5. Let brownies cool slightly, then spread peanut butter on top while still warm.

## Additional Notes

» Optional: add unsweetened coconut flakes, slivered almonds, or chopped walnuts on top with a small dollop of sugar-free whipped topping.

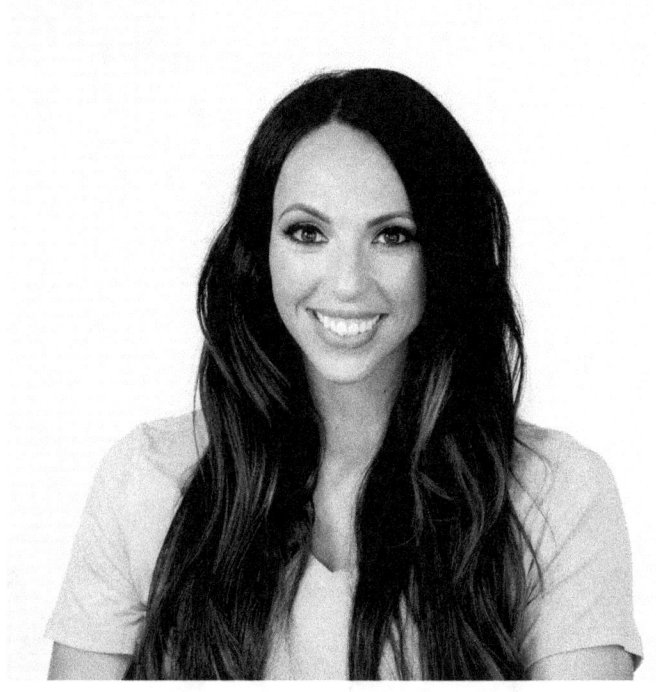

## *About The Author*

Kristy Jo Wengert is a certified Fitness Nutrition Specialist, Weight Loss Specialist, Personal Trainer, and author of the Power Foods Lifestyle nutrition line. After overcoming over 15 years of disordered eating and exercising as well as a chronic pain condition due to three lateral curves in her spine, she is now on a mission to help as many people who will listen to her strategic approach to health and a higher daily quality of life. Her work has been featured on KUTV 2News, the Matt Townsend Show, and numerous podcasts and radio interviews. She is the host of the Power Foods Lifestyle podcast and has coached over 5,000 women to healthier body composition and mindsets around their bodies.

www.ingramcontent.com/pod-product-compliance
Lightning Source LLC
Chambersburg PA
CBHW052116110526
**44592CB00013B/1630**